THE HUNDRED-YEAR LIE

RANDALL FITZGERALD has written investigative features for *The Washington Post* and *The Wall Street Journal*, and for twenty years was a contributing editor for *Reader's Digest*, where he researched, wrote, and edited articles on science and medicine. The author of six previous books, he lives in northern California.

Praise for *The Hundred-Year Lie*

"Well-crafted and thought-provoking."   —*Library Journal*

"One of the most interesting books of 2006. . . . Fitzgerald fearlessly challenges our poisonous penchant for ingesting processed foods, polluted waters, and modern medications."   —BookLovers Review

"Challenges several myths established and perpetuated by the food, pharmaceutical, and chemical industries, points out government's failure to better protect consumers, and offers suggestions for restoring a more healthful and less toxic society."   —*Burlington County Times*

"A devastating exposé of how chemicals in everyday products are polluting our physical bodies."   —*Arizona Networking News*

"This is a must-read for anyone truly interested in a healthier life."
                    —Book Sense

"Read *The Hundred-Year Lie* by Randall Fitzgerald if you were impressed by Al Gore's *An Inconvenient Truth*."   —BlogforAmerica.com

ALSO BY RANDALL FITZGERALD

Lucky You!
Mugged by the State
Cosmic Test Tube
When Government Goes Private
Porkbarrel (with Gerald Lipson)
The Complete Book of Extraterrestrial Encounters

THE HUNDRED-YEAR LIE

HOW TO PROTECT YOURSELF FROM THE CHEMICALS THAT ARE DESTROYING YOUR HEALTH

RANDALL FITZGERALD

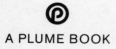
A PLUME BOOK

PLUME
Published by Penguin Group
Penguin Group (USA) Inc., 375 Hudson Street, New York, New York 10014, U.S.A. • Penguin
Group (Canada), 90 Eglinton Avenue East, Suite 700, Toronto, Ontario, Canada M4P 2Y3 (a division of Pearson Penguin Canada Inc.) • Penguin Books Ltd., 80 Strand, London WC2R 0RL, England • Penguin Ireland, 25 St. Stephen's Green, Dublin 2, Ireland (a division of Penguin Books Ltd.)
Penguin Group (Australia), 250 Camberwell Road, Camberwell, Victoria 3124, Australia (a division of Pearson Australia Group Pty. Ltd.) • Penguin Books India Pvt. Ltd., 11 Community Centre,
Panchsheel Park, New Delhi – 110 017, India • Penguin Group (NZ), 67 Apollo Drive, Rosedale,
North Shore 0745, Auckland, New Zealand (a division of Pearson New Zealand Ltd.) • Penguin
Books (South Africa) (Pty.) Ltd., 24 Sturdee Avenue, Rosebank, Johannesburg 2196, South Africa

Penguin Books Ltd., Registered Offices: 80 Strand, London WC2R 0RL, England

Published by Plume, a member of Penguin Group (USA) Inc. Previously published in a Dutton
edition.

First Plume Printing, July 2007
10 9 8 7 6 5 4 3 2 1

Copyright © Randall Fitzgerald, 2006
All rights reserved

Ⓟ REGISTERED TRADEMARK—MARCA REGISTRADA

The Library of Congress has catalogued the Dutton edition as follows:
Fitzgerald, Randall.
    The hundred-year lie : how food and medicine are destroying your health / Randall Fitzgerald.
        p. cm.
    ISBN 0-525-94951-8 (hc.)
    ISBN 978-0-452-28839-3 (pbk.)
    1. Toxicology—Popular works. 2. Food—Toxicology—Popular works. 3. Drugs—Toxicology—
Popular works. 4. Drugs—Side effects—Popular works. 5. Pharmaceutical industry—Corrupt
Practices—United States—Popular works. 6. Food industry—Corrupt practices—United States—
Popular works. 7. Alternative medicine—Popular works. I. Title.
    RA1213.F58 2006
    615.9—dc22   2005037244

Printed in the United States of America

CONTENTS

THE HUNDRED-YEAR LIE

INTRODUCTION

WHAT ARE WE DOING TO OURSELVES?

Over the past one hundred years, our species has been engaged in a vast and complicated chemistry experiment. Each and every one of us, along with our children, our parents, and our grandparents, has been a guinea pig in this experiment, which uses our bodies, our health, our wealth, and our goodwill to test the proposition that modern science can improve upon the foods and medicines of nature.

My awareness of what I will refer to on these pages as the Hundred-Year Lie came about gradually from a concern for members of my family who seemed to be on a slippery slope of health dilemmas. My younger brother had become overweight, apparently from the side effects of prescription drug use and a diet of processed foods. The excess weight facilitated the onset of type 2 diabetes, a diagnosis prompting physicians to prescribe still more drugs for his daily consumption. My father took the prescription drug Vioxx for arthritis and suffered a stroke, becoming one of thousands of people apparently victimized by this drug before it was withdrawn from the market as a health danger. Both my father and mother take more than a half dozen prescription drugs every day for various ailments ranging from thyroid imbalance to high blood pressure. Some of these drugs were prescribed to counteract the side effects of the other medications. Their total monthly cost of nine hundred dollars exceeds what my parents spend on food.

My sister had her uterus removed, at age forty-one, as a result of fibroid tumors. These tumors erupted a few months following the steroid injections she had received as treatment for a car accident injury. She has numerous female friends in her age group who have also had hysterectomies. Others have been found to be infertile. "If this trend continues," she remarked to me after her surgery in 2005, "we may poison ourselves to extinction, and I mean that literally."

Among my friends and acquaintances, all of whom are baby boomers like me, or younger, three are battling various forms of cancer, three others are in remission from cancer, two have come down with multiple sclerosis, one man and one woman have AIDS, two people suffer from Parkinson's disease in its advanced stages, two in their thirties have Crohn's disease, and three others endure such severe bouts of migraines and food allergies that doctors say, only half-jokingly, they must be "allergic to civilization."

The synergy of imbalances in my own circle of friends mirrors the larger patterns at work throughout our culture. During the three decades I spent as an investigative reporter for newspapers and magazines, my journalistic survival often depended on an ability to recognize patterns in the activities of people, government, and businesses. Sometimes these patterns and trends could only be discerned if I visualized the broader historical context. To achieve that detachment and overview, I would pretend that I was a stranger in a strange land, an alien visiting this planet and this culture to see if anything made sense.

The patterns and observations you are about to confront may seem so alien and alarming, so contrary to your comforting worldview, that you too may feel like a stranger in your own strange land. But please don't let this warning dissuade you from venturing forward. We all periodically need such jolts to awaken us to a larger web of truths that we have overlooked or chosen to ignore.

Like many people, I have mostly taken food and health for granted, at least until a medical crisis intervened to remind me that I am subject to the laws of nature. Once the crisis passes, once medical technology treats my symptoms (or doesn't), I return slowly but surely to my old habits of thoughtless eating and reflexive consumption.

During the research for this book I began to see patterns etched in the mounting body of evidence that, despite our remarkable sophistication in medical technology that keeps the seriously ill alive and extends life spans, our overall health condition as a society has degenerated alarmingly and rapidly. Over the past one hundred years our cancer mortality rate has gone from 3 percent of all deaths to 20 percent of all deaths. Our incidence of diabetes went from 0.1 percent of the population to almost 20 percent. Heart disease went from being almost nonexistent to killing more than seven hundred thousand people a year. At the same time, health care costs have risen until the United States now spends twice as much on medicine and care per person per year than any other industrialized nation in the world.

What further jolted me into an awareness of the perils we face from our food, our medicine, and our health choices was a series of news stories that normally I would have overlooked, as many of you probably did, if only because the drumbeat of alarming headlines often feels overwhelming and beyond our control. This time, however, I paid close attention to how these news reports, appearing in the span of a few weeks in 2004, brought the slippery slope and our position on it into sharper focus.

In the first report, based on a study from the science journal *Public Health*, I learned that the incidence of death from brain diseases, such as Alzheimer's, Parkinson's, and motor neuron disorders, was found to have tripled in nine Western countries, including the United States, during the period of 1974 to 1997. The most likely causes researchers identified were exposure to pesticides sprayed on crops, synthetic chemicals from the processed foods that we consume, and industrial chemicals used in almost every aspect of our modern lives. "There's no single cause," admitted Colin Pritchard, one of the British authors of the study. "Most of the time we have no studies on all the multiple interactions of the chemical combinations."

Food seemed to be a major culprit for this toxicity, because Japan, alone among the ten countries studied, experienced no increase in brain disease mortality, apparently as a result of the Japanese diet being healthier than Western diets. When Japanese citizens relocate to Western countries and consume processed foods, their disease rates exceed those of Japan as a whole.

A day after reading this report I heard a radio show during which a California state environmental official made this startling claim: Recent water testing had showed that 60 percent of the rivers and streams in that state contained high levels of Prozac, Ritalin, and antibiotics. How could such contamination possibly have happened? Because people had dumped their excess prescription drugs into those bodies of water or had flushed them directly or through bodily waste into sewer and septic systems, where the chemicals then leeched into groundwater. I had to wonder what effects those drugs were having on fish and other wildlife and what levels of toxins might be accumulating in the tissues of people who consume the contaminated fish.

Several days passed, and I came across another, even more disturbing report. American supermarket foods are polluted with toxic chemical flame retardants. (Yes, you read that correctly!) A fire-retardant chemical with the acronym of PBDE, used in carpeting, electronics, and furniture, is being absorbed by the fatty tissues of animals. Processed into food, these animal products have contaminated thirty-one of thirty-two common name-brand groceries found in a representative sampling of the nation's supermarkets. That finding emerged in the peer-reviewed science journal *Environmental Science & Technology*, based on a survey and chemical analysis of thirty-two products, including ice cream, eggs, milk, butter, cheese, chicken, and turkey. Only nonfat milk contained no PBDE molecules in detectable levels. Once in the human body, PBDE can persist in our tissues for years, maybe a lifetime. No one has yet studied what levels of PBDE are harmful to humans. But animal tests have found the chemical to be carcinogenic and damaging to the nervous system, hormonal functions, and the reproductive organs.

After a little more digging I found a study sponsored by the National Oceanic and Atmospheric Administration that described how PBDE was concentrated in sediment hundreds of feet down in Lake Michigan. Fish have been absorbing the PBDE into their fatty tissues and passing the chemical on to humans who eat the fish. "These chemicals are showing up all over the world," warned Bill Sonzogni, a University of Wisconsin scientist who helped draft the study. "The Great Lakes—because of the food chain for bioconcentrating contaminants—sometimes serves as a sentinel for other parts of the world." (Bioconcentration means fish absorb the toxins, and when humans eat the fish, these toxins accumulate in their fatty tissues.)

Another report that surfaced from Britain tested how toxic human body tissues have become. Researchers with the World Wildlife Fund (WWF) conducted extensive blood testing on seven families and detected at least seventy-five synthetic chemicals in the bodies of the parents and their children, including pesticides and PCBs from electrical equipment.

A nine-year-old farm boy from Wales, Alwyn Jones, was found to be contaminated with twenty-nine separate toxic chemicals, despite having been born years after several of the chemicals had been outlawed as health threats. Alwyn's mother, Enid, who registered twenty-one toxic chemicals in her body, handled the news philosophically: "It just shows we are exposed to such a variety of manmade chemicals. It is a lottery as to how many we have in our bodies and at what rate these are building up in our children. It worries me that we don't know enough about what is in the products we use in our homes and their potential health effects."

Subsequent studies have expanded the scope of concern. Medical researchers at the Mount Sinai School of Medicine in New York found an average of ninety-one industrial compounds, pollutants, and other synthetic chemicals in the blood and urine of nine volunteers who had no occupational or geographical connection to these chemicals or where they are manufactured. More than half of these chemicals are known to be responsible for birth defects, cancer, or brain and nervous system disorders in humans. An even more extensive round of testing by the Centers for Disease Control and Prevention, involving 2,400 adults and children, documented more than two hundred synthetic chemical toxins in the subjects' bodies, with hundreds more chemicals suspected to be present.

"An effect of this contamination is that we are now one of the most polluted species on the face of this planet," contends Paula Baillie-Hamilton, an Oxford-educated physician in Britain who is one of the leading authorities on toxins in food. "Indeed, we are all so contaminated that if we were cannibals our meat would be banned from human consumption."

How did we become so toxic? What thrust us as a culture and as individuals onto this slippery slope? How can we navigate our way back to a healthier and less toxic future? These were some of the questions that haunted me as I undertook the research for this book.

THE SYNTHETICS BELIEF SYSTEM

What links all of the preceding stories and studies and levels of toxicity is a belief system that emerged during the twentieth century. Some call it a better life through chemistry. I have labeled it the Hundred-Year Lie. The lie really began in earnest in 1906, the year the U.S. Congress enacted the Pure Foods and Drugs Act, the first law of its kind that gave the public a false sense of security about the safety of its foods and medicines. As we observe the centennial of this law, it is worth putting the belief system it spawned into some historical perspective.

The synthetics revolution is a by-product of activities within three sectors of the U.S. economy—the processed foods industry, the pharmaceutical industry, and the chemical industry. These economic interests influence our diet and health from the womb to the grave. The control we give them over our lives springs directly from our acceptance of this belief system's primary conceit: their lab-created synthetics are as benign as—and more effective than—naturally occurring foods and medicines. That claim is what I describe as the Hundred-Year Lie.

Our indoctrination into the synthetics mythology has its deeper roots in an awestruck fealty to science and technology, whose powers have simultaneously blessed us and blinded us. We live in a prosperous system where the economic principles of supply and demand, competitive markets, and profit motives relentlessly drive the industrialization of our food, medicine, and health care. This system has created cheaper and more plentiful food and produced a host of medical technologies that may save lives and extend lives in almost miraculous ways (if we can afford them). But what have we overlooked, what have we sacrificed, in return?

In our food choices, we seem to have traded the safety of our long-term health for lower prices and convenience, though even the cost incentive may actually be an illusion, given the medical bills a diet of processed foods may eventually generate. This book will show that the sheer proliferation of processed food products (more than three hundred thousand currently on store shelves), prescription drugs (more than thirty thousand available), and nonprescription drugs (at least two hundred thousand brands) constitutes an inherently toxic synergy. We have introduced thousands of chemicals into our diet. How will they each affect us? And how will they react with one another inside our bodies? The study of synergy—the ways in which chemicals may react in unexpected ways—is a new field in which researchers are now making alarming discoveries. Lace our food and medicine with the toxic brew of synthetic chemicals that now percolate through every aspect of our natural environment and we have a recipe for massive immune system breakdown and a health-care system disaster.

The fundamental premise on which modern medicine was founded, the Hippocratic oath (with its edict to do no harm), no longer seems to motivate the provision of our drugs or our medical care, except perhaps as an afterthought to avoid lawsuits. Consider just a representative sampling of the findings collected from reputable sources about what is really in our food, water, vitamins, prescription drugs, childhood vaccines, cosmetics, and in our homes.

- When you read "made with natural flavors" on a food label, you are probably being deceived, because natural flavors and artificial flavors usually contain the same synthetic chemicals.
- In large feedlots, 100 percent of the cattle are fed five or more sex hormones, such as progesterone and testosterone, to accelerate weight gain, and these hormones are known to cause reproductive dysfunction and cancers in humans.
- Many of our commercial dairy and meat products come from animals that consumed livestock feed made from the remains of tens of millions of dogs and cats that were killed with euthanasia drugs at animal shelters and veterinary clinics.
- Medical evidence is emerging that suggests that the artificial sweeteners in diet soft drinks may cause brain tumors and neurological diseases, such as Parkinson's and Alzheimer's. The occurrence of these diseases has risen dramatically, in proportion with the expanded use of those synthetic sweeteners.
- At least 70 percent of the processed foods in your local grocery store contain at least one genetically engineered ingredient that has never been tested for its potential harm.
- More than three thousand synthetic chemicals are regularly

added to U.S. food products, and hardly any have been tested for their synergistic (interactive) toxin-producing effects in the human body.

- Most vitamins and supplements sold in the United States that are advertised as natural are actually synthetic chemical concoctions that contain coal tar, preservatives, artificial colorings, and a vast range of other potentially harmful additives.
- More than twenty-five thousand chemicals are in the cosmetics sold in the United States, yet less than 4 percent of these ingredients have ever been tested for toxicity and safety.
- Within the nine or so vaccines given your children before they enter school are additives and preservatives, including mercury, aluminum, MSG, formaldehyde, and others linked to disorders ranging from brain and nerve damage to autism and attention deficit disorder.

Many people want to believe that the U.S. Food and Drug Administration protects them from anything dangerous in our drug or food supplies. The fact is that when the FDA approves a new drug for public use it has *not* studied that drug's safety. The agency relies upon safety information from the drug manufacturers to make its approval decisions. Nor does the FDA test the safety of ingredients in cosmetics and personal-care products.

Chemical companies create and inject so many hundreds of new synthetic chemicals into our lives each year that regulatory agencies and toxicologists can no longer even find the time or resources to develop new tests to detect their presence in our bodies or in the environment.

Physicians can't protect us either. A medical journal study found that 44 percent of drug advertising in medical journals, and 42 percent of drug information given doctors by drug company representatives, would lead physicians to improperly prescribe medications to their patients. More than 100,000 people in the United States die every year from adverse reactions to their prescription drugs and more than two million people a year have serious but nonfatal reactions, claims the American Medical Association.

For the first time in human history, we are tinkering with the developmental cycle of our species by taking short-sighted actions that, while intended to advance civilization, could actually threaten its very survival.

We are on a slippery slope of redefining what it means to be "normal" or even human.

CHOOSING NATURAL ALTERNATIVES

Throughout my professional life, I have written and spoken favorably about maximizing individual freedom in all aspects of life, including free markets and free enterprise. The bedrock of my libertarian perspective has always been the idea that as individuals, our freedom to choose is dependent upon a right to treat our bodies as private property that we own and control. In that spirit I believe we each should have a private property right to keep our bodies free from trespass by toxins. Our private property rights should extend to keeping the air our bodies breathe clear of toxins, the water we drink free of toxins, the food we eat clean of toxins.

While we may never be able to totally eliminate our risk of exposure to harmful toxins, we can manage those risks and reduce our chances of harm. The future of food, nutrition, and health is about empowering ourselves as sovereign individuals. To accomplish that, to make informed decisions and choices, we all need the freedom of access to relevant information about the quality and purity of what our body absorbs.

Freedom to choose represents a shift in consciousness toward self-diagnosis, a wider range of medical choices, and natural approaches to food, health, and healing. This new system is what I call the *naturally occurring paradigm*—it is about empowering our immune systems the natural way, using food as nature intended, to help protect ourselves from illness and disease.

For many of us, before we can discover natural healing alternatives, we must first experience the desperation of having exhausted the entire range of synthetic chemical remedies offered by modern Western medicine. What happened to me personally, though my ailment was minor compared to most, still serves to dramatize the limitations of our reliance on synthetic drugs.

While on a journalistic assignment in South Dakota, I slipped and fell during a snowstorm. When I hit the street curb, I took the full force of impact on the right side of my lower back. The next day, my injury and pain were exacerbated by a cramped three-hour flight home to California. The throbbing sensation in my lower back became so severe that my body began slipping into shock.

Friends rushed me to the emergency room of a hospital, where I was hooked up to an intravenous morphine drip. The morphine barely dulled my sensation of pain. X-rays for broken bones were negative, and an attending physician speculated that the fall had bruised one of my kidneys. He wrote me a prescription for a strong narcotic painkiller and sent me home with the confession, "There is nothing else that can be done for you." The emergency room visit cost seven hundred dollars, which came out of my own pocket since my insurance policy had a thousand-dollar deductible.

Though I debated whether to fill the prescription because of my concern about the narcotic's potential for disorientation and addiction, the discomfort was so constant and intense, magnified by my every movement, that I could not imagine I had any other choice.

As I walked in agonizing pain to a neighborhood pharmacy, I happened to pass by a chiropractic clinic. Though I had no reason to believe that a chiropractor could provide relief, my intuition urged me to at least inquire. A middle-aged chiropractor tended to me immediately and applied a heat compress to my lower back, followed by an ultrasound treatment. She then spent ten minutes doing deep tissue massage on the affected area. She explained how these manipulations combined with heat and sound—a synergistic effect—would help to restore the internal alignment of my kidney.

Her technique worked like magic. I got off the table and my pain was instantly and completely gone, and it never returned. The session only cost fifty-five dollars, and the experience sold me on the idea that the synergistic effects of natural treatments and remedies can be effective and economical.

HOLDING OURSELVES ACCOUNTABLE

This book is intended to be a wake-up call that inspires action and accountability on your part, not a gloom-and-doom attempt to immobilize you with fear. It will offer tried and proven food and medicine alternatives to synthetic chemicals.

My hope is that this book becomes a step in the education process that will help to lift the fog of confusion we find ourselves in. We do have a choice about whether we will be a victim or not. We can view ourselves as an individual market; a consumer market that we own and control. Or we can allow our food and medicine and product-ingredient choices to be made for us by institutions that regard us as little more than interchangeable parts of an economic engine. If we fail to exercise our freedom in daily food and health choices, we affect not only our own well-being but the well-being of those we care about and who depend upon us for good judgment.

Effective natural-health solutions *do* exist, and they are rooted in ancient traditions that are our legacy. Thousands of years of trial and error, of human intuition and observation being tested and retested through the generations, confirm the existence of a veritable Garden of Eden of naturally occurring abundance for our well-being.

Some general, commonsense truths emerged from my research:

—*Not* all synthetics, at least as far as we know, are toxic to us.
—*Not* all naturally occurring substances from nature are benign.

However, broadly speaking, the evidence indicates that most naturally occurring foods and medicines are healthy for us, as they have been for our species for thousands of years, while many if not most synthetic chemicals in foods and medicines pose some health risk.

Exposure to a few toxic substances, or to a wide range of molecules from a variety of synthetics, may not trigger illness or disease in you. But then again, it might. Medical science simply cannot predict who is susceptible to which chemicals, at which dosage levels, or how additive effects and synergies create toxic conditions in the human body. These risk-factor uncertainties during the normal course of our lives constitute a form of biological Russian roulette that each of us plays with our bodies every day based on our food, medicine, and environmental choices.

We cannot expect to totally eliminate these risk factors, at least not in our lifetimes. Chemical toxins respect no boundaries and trespass against us whenever we breathe or drink or eat. Our only reasonable hope is to learn how to limit our risks and manage our exposure to synthetic toxins so that we might increase our chances of leading healthy lives.

All that I ask of you the reader is that you pretend you are a stranger in a strange land. Pretend that you are being confronted for the first time by the evidence of what a century of human efforts has accomplished in trying to improve upon the intelligence of nature while ignoring nature's inherent wisdom.

Let me tell you the story of the Hundred-Year Lie.

PART ONE

DOWN THE RABBIT HOLE

Our Vicious Cycle

We are surrounded every day by an invisible sea of synthetic chemicals, and our bodies absorb them like sponges until we are toxic.

We consume foods that have been depleted of essential natural healing nutrients. These nutrients have been replaced by synthetic chemical additives.

These additives in our processed foods interact synergistically in our bodies with synthetic chemicals absorbed from our water, our air, and our consumer products, weakening our immune systems.

Once weakened, we become susceptible to illnesses and diseases that medical practitioners treat with synthetic chemical drug compounds that often prove even more toxic to us.

And this cycle in our culture and in our lives repeats itself over and over. . . .

CHAPTER ONE

READING THE SIGNS

"Today we are witnessing another medical anomaly—a unique pattern of illness involving chemically exposed people who subsequently report multisystem symptoms and new-onset chemical and food intolerances. These intolerances may be the hallmark for a new disease process, just as fever is a hallmark for infection."

—Dr. Claudia Miller of the University of Texas
Health Science Center, writing in *Annals of the New York
Academy of Sciences*, 2001

About the size of a magazine, the sign has black lettering on a white background and can be found posted at eye level just inches from Wal-Mart's main entrance:

**WARNING: Products Sold Or Used On These Premises
May Contain Chemicals Known To The State Of
California To Cause Cancer, Birth Defects,
Or Other Reproductive Harm.**

Wal-Mart shoppers are surging past the sign, and I notice that no one ever glances at it. After fifteen minutes of watching people ignore the sign as if it doesn't exist or else has nothing to do with them, I decide to conduct an informal survey.

When a thirty-something lady approaches with two young children, I beckon to her, "Excuse me, what do you think this sign means?"

Her eyes follow my finger to the bold-lettered words.

"It's a liability thing," she replies after a quick read. "In case someone gets sick inside and tries to sue the store."

She resumes her march, pulling both kids along.

"But wait!" I call after her. "Could it be too dangerous to go inside?"

Her head swivels around with irritation. "I shop here all the time! If there was any danger, someone would tell us!"

"Maybe that's what they're doing with the sign," I respond, but too late. She is already charging through the automatic doors and headed for the inner sanctum of consumerism.

I ask a clerk inside if I can speak with a store manager. She directs me to an affable, rosy-cheeked woman in her mid-forties named Marilee, the customer service manager. Describing myself as a customer, I inquire what the sign outside the front door means. At first she doesn't know what I am talking about. After I recite what the sign says, suddenly it dawns on her.

"Oh right, there is a sign. It's because we sell products in here that contain harmful chemicals."

"Should I be concerned about coming in?" I ask.

"Oh, it's not in the air or anything. The state of California just requires us to warn people."

She seems puzzled when I continue showing interest and asking questions. She professes that she can't recall any customer wanting to know about the sign before.

"Can you tell me, what are the harmful chemicals?"

She thinks for a moment before slowly shaking her head. "No, I can't. Why don't you consult our Web site. It has everything you need to know."

She is misinformed. After a half hour searching the Wal-Mart Web site, I discover it contains no information about anything other than products and services, so I shoot off an e-mail with my sign questions to Wal-Mart's corporate office. My e-mail produces a telephone call several days later from an executive identifying himself as Mark. (Everyone seems to use only first names at Wal-Mart.)

"The sign is a federal mandate but state regulated," explains Mark, who has about the most cheerful and courteous voice I have ever heard.

"So, does the state or the stores do any air quality tests inside to detect toxic fumes or chemical synergies?"

"Why, no," replies Mark, still cheerful. "Other than the ventilating systems, no one does any monitoring of the air inside our stores at all."

Before we hang up Mark promises to look for the list of harmful chemicals and contact me again. (I am still waiting!) Then he makes a confession: "By the way, you're the first customer I know of who has contacted us about that sign."

"Why do you think that is?" I reply.

Mark laughs. "People only seem to read a sign if there's a price tag on it."

As I later discover, the sign is mandated by Proposition 65, a state initiative passed by California voters in 1986, requiring businesses to post warnings if their premises contain dangerous chemicals. A state government agency, the Office of Environmental Health Hazard Assessment, every year updates its list of chemicals in public use that are known to cause cancer, birth defects, or other reproductive harm. That list now exceeds 750 chemicals and includes additives and ingredients in food, drugs, pesticides, solvents, and a range of common household products.

Walking into any Wal-Mart store today, or for that matter any Kmart or Target or similar business, provides us with a museum-quality tour of the synthetics belief system that evolved over the past century. We are confronted by tens of thousands of products containing synthetic chemicals. Many are releasing molecules into the air, a process called off-gassing. Practically every label we read on every product we pick up contains a list of chemical names that to most of us sound about as comprehensible as ancient Greek.

We either take an "ignorance is bliss" attitude about these chemicals, or we adopt a faith-based mind-set that assumes some agency of the federal or state government, or the product manufacturers themselves, will warn us of any health dangers. But even when such warnings are posted, as with the Wal-Mart sign, we nonchalantly go about our daily lives pretending that what we don't know won't hurt us.

Let's examine the reality of what we confront on a daily basis. If you are a typical person, on any normal morning of your life the following routine should be similar to your experience. You awaken from sleeping on a mattress that was coated with flame-retardant chemicals during its manufacture—as most mattresses are—and which emits minuscule amounts of formaldehyde gas and a brominated substance known to be carcinogenic, which your body readily absorbs. You pad on your bare feet toward the bathroom, across a synthetic carpet treated—as most carpets are during manufacture—with benzene and styrene and several other cancer-causing chemicals.

Once in the bathroom, you turn on the faucet and splash your face with tap water laced with fluoride and chlorine, both carcinogens (most tap water also contains traces of herbicides and pharmaceutical drugs). You open a plastic bottle of Listerine mouthwash (or a similar brand) and gargle, not realizing that the plastic bottle has leached its own chemicals into a mouthwash mixture that already includes four active ingredients along with a half dozen flavoring and coloring chemicals. If you read the mouthwash label you will find the following: "WARNINGS: Do not administer to children under twelve years of age. Do not swallow. In case of accidental ingestion, seek professional assistance or contact a Poison Control Center immediately." You pick up your Crest toothpaste and find it also has a warning label: "If more than used for brushing is accidentally swallowed, get medical help. . . ." Though sodium fluoride is the only "active" ingredient listed on this toothpaste container, there are other chemicals in this concoction that don't have to be revealed to you, because they are classified as "inert" and are thus protected under trade secrecy laws.

You raise your arms and apply Speed Stick deodorant, which contains seven chemicals, including aluminum, parabens (a preservative), propylene glycol (a lubricant and suspected cancer agent), and other chemicals disguised under "fragrance," which is another trade secrecy term. On average, according to the FDA, we each use nine personal-care products daily, containing about 126 chemical ingredients. If you use body lotions, they contain penetration-enhancing chemicals that can drive toxins from other toiletries deeper into your flesh. Before leaving the bathroom you pull a prescription drug (with a warning label attached) out of the medicine cabinet and swallow this mixture of synthetic chemicals. All the while you have been breathing benzene fumes (capable of causing leukemia) from that deodorizer you installed under the commode seat lid.

Back in your bedroom you pull on clothes fresh from the dry cleaner and expose yourself to fumes and residues of trichloroethylene and n-hexane, chemicals known to cause nerve cell damage, memory loss, and cardiac abnormalities. If you have mothballs in your closet, you are exposing yourself to the carcinogenic pesticide dichlorobenzene, which is also found in toilet deodorizers. If your clothing contains synthetic fibers, you are being exposed to a form of plastic, and the newer the clothing, the more it off-gases molecules of plasticizer fumes. Your clothes may also contain flame-retardant chemicals that are notorious releasers of toxic fumes. The more tightly insulated your bedroom and the other rooms of your dwelling, the greater the outgas collection effect of the chemicals from your furniture, wall paint, rugs, and carpeting, and the greater the impact on your brain, with symptoms like mood swings, feelings of spaciness, headaches, and an inability to concentrate.

You walk into your kitchen and pour yourself a bowl of cereal containing nearly a dozen synthetic chemical food additives, including the sweetener aspartame, which has been linked to a wide range of allergies and illnesses. Meanwhile, while eating you turn on the dishwasher and expose yourself to a cloud of chlorine fumes. You fix yourself a sandwich you will eat for lunch later at work. You use meat that contains nitrates, synthetic hormones, and antibiotics that were injected into the animals when they were alive. You place lettuce and sliced tomato on top, each of which contains the residues of a half dozen different pesticides. Then you wrap the sandwich in Saran Wrap (or a similar brand of plastic), which contains vinyl chloride, a carcinogen known to cause liver, brain, and lung cancers. As you are preparing this meal, fumes from the toxic bug spray and the cleaning solvents beneath your sink (all with warning labels attached) are further contaminating the air you breathe.

Here we are barely into the first hour of your day, you haven't even left your home yet, and already you've been absorbing molecules from hundreds of synthetic chemicals. You haven't even come in contact yet with the really harsh toxins that lurk outside, generated by car exhaust and manufacturing processes, or that lie in wait for you at your workplace and in the fast food and junk food that you sometimes consume.

"We are the first generation of people to ever be exposed on a daily basis to such an unprecedented number of chemicals," says Dr. Sherry A. Rogers, a fellow of the American College of Allergy and Immunology. "At no other time have patients, through reading and education, had such an important and crucial role in determining their own wellness."

MYTHS WE CHERISH

TOXICITY IS SOMEONE ELSE'S PROBLEM

While it may sound rather harsh to label each and every one of us a living toxic waste dump, the reality of the body burden of toxins we each bear does support that description. We absorb so many synthetic chemicals during an average lifetime that, according to some reports, when we die our bodies decompose more slowly today than if we had died just three decades ago.

Five major public surveys testing blood and urine for chemical contamination have been conducted among thousands of volunteers, with results indicating that every resident of industrialized countries now carries within his or her body an average of seven hundred synthetic chemicals absorbed from our food, water, and air. The actual number of chemicals constituting our body burden is probably much higher, because some toxins are embedded deep in organs and tissues. A toxicologist's ability to detect chemical toxins depends on knowing what to look for, and every time they devise a new test, they tend to find evidence for the presence of more toxic invaders.

In 2001, scientists at the U.S. Centers for Disease Control and Prevention in Atlanta surveyed 2,400 people and searched for 148 specific toxic compounds in their blood and urine. Every single test subject's body contained dozens of these toxins. Children were found to be carrying bigger doses of the chemicals than adults, especially a class of chemicals called pyrethroids—found in most household pesticides—and phthalates, a group of chemicals distributed widely in plastics and cosmetics, primarily nail polish.

Environment ministers from thirteen European Union countries had their blood tested at an international health conference in 2004 and were horrified to discover that every one of them had been contaminated by synthetic chemicals from pizza packaging, pesticides, plastics, fragrances, and industrial solvents. At least twenty-two chemicals banned in Europe during the 1970s still turned up in the blood samples of these government officials.

In response to these studies, the American Chemistry Council, representing the U.S. chemical manufacturing industry, issued a press release stating "the mere detection of a chemical does not necessarily indicate a risk to health." It didn't consider these reports to be a cause for undue concern. This attitude characterizes one of the myths that we as a culture tell ourselves. When we don't like the evidence of what is happening to us, we redefine what is normal. So now it is considered normal and not a cause for concern that we carry around inside of us hundreds of potentially toxic synthetic chemicals that have never been inside of human beings before the twentieth century?

As a challenge to the chemical industry, a study was done by an organization called the Environmental Working Group that used two testing laboratories to measure chemical toxins in the umbilical-cord blood of ten randomly chosen babies born in August and September of 2004 in U.S. hospitals. An average of two hundred synthetic chemicals were detected, which means these ten babies were exposed to an onslaught of toxins from their mothers during a critical developmental phase before birth. Synthetics in their blood included eight perfluorochemicals used as stain and oil repellants in fast food packaging, dozens of flame retardants and pesticides, and the Teflon chemical PFOA. Nearly all of the toxins have been linked to cancer, brain and nervous system disorders, birth defects, or developmental problems. Should we consider that body burden being carried by fetuses as normal?

Because our planet is bathed in a synthetic chemical soup and the toxic molecules travel widely by attaching themselves to dust particles blowing in wind currents, no human being or food supply anywhere, no matter how remote, is immune to being contaminated. In Arctic Circle wilderness villages, the Inuit mothers now carry such huge loads of PCBs and mercury in their bodies that their breast milk would be categorized as hazardous waste by the Food and Drug Administration if it were being evaluated for human consumption.

"Arctic people and animals are hundreds of miles from any significant source of pollution, living in one of the most desolate spots on the planet, yet, paradoxically, they are among the planet's most contaminated living organisms," writes *Los Angeles Times* reporter Marla Cone in her 2005 book, *Silent Snow: The Slow Poisoning of the Arctic.* "The Arctic's people and animals have been transformed into living, deep-freeze archives storing toxic memories of the industrialized world's past and present." (Molecules of toxic chemicals attach themselves to dust particles and travel the upper air currents north, to where colder climates draw them like a magnet.)

Cone identified at least two hundred synthetic chemicals that are adversely affecting the health of indigenous people at the top of the world. Children in this region suffer extremely high rates of infectious diseases apparently brought on by a suppression of their immune systems from exposure to chemical toxins. Similar effects are showing up in animal populations in the form of viral epidemics.

A favorable review of Cone's book in *The San Francisco Chronicle* summarized the challenge that her findings pose for us: ". . . as more chemicals are being developed and marketed without sufficient toxicity testing—as more lawn products, pesticides and flame retardants, to name a few household culprits, are being spewed into the environment—it becomes increasingly urgent that every single person living in an industrialized nation learn what Greenlander Ingmar Egede already knows: 'The chemical threat is the ultimate threat to mankind, worse than bombs and war. You cannot hide from it. It reaches everywhere in the world.' "

MYTHS WE CHERISH

THE GOVERNMENT KNOWS WHAT IS SAFE

No one knows exactly how many synthetic chemicals have been unleashed on this planet. A generally accepted figure—necessarily an estimate—is that one hundred thousand are in use worldwide, with more than one thousand new chemicals entering the marketplace every year. The United

States Environmental Protection Agency keeps a list of about eighty-five thousand in its registry, and of these only a small fraction have ever been tested individually for their impact on the health of human beings. Many fewer still have been tested for their additive or synergistic, multiple-interaction impacts on health.

Toxins expert Doris J. Rapp warns us that the rules have been written in such a way that we can never know what is safe until people or animals in the wild begin suffering. "The Toxic Substances Control Act of 1976 allows chemicals to be sold and used unless they are proven to be a risk. The EPA, however, does not conduct its own safety tests, but relies on research conducted by manufacturers. Yes, you read it correctly. Is the fox in charge of designing the chicken coop?"

Over the past three decades, chemical companies have provided the EPA with health data for only about 15 percent of the tens of thousands of new synthetic chemicals that have been introduced into the marketplace, according to a 2005 report by the Government Accountability Office, the investigative arm of the U.S. Congress. "EPA does not routinely assess existing chemicals, has limited information on their health and environmental risks, and has issued few regulations controlling such chemicals," the report charged.

When it comes to chemicals added to cosmetics and many other personal-care products, the FDA knows as much about their safety as you do. Under FDA regulations neither cosmetic products nor cosmetic ingredients are reviewed or approved by the FDA before they are sold to the public. Every consumer uses an average of nine personal-care products containing 126 separate ingredients each day, estimates the Environmental Working Group, and at least one-third of these ingredients have been identified as causing cancer or other serious health problems.

What distresses and perplexes me is the realization that even if government had the resources to thoroughly conduct widespread safety testing—which it doesn't—our technology is too primitive to detect all of the synthetic chemicals in combination or to complete the task within our own lifetimes or even within the life spans of any of our grandchildren.

Considering the enormity of this challenge, Sheldon Krimsky, in his 2000 book, *Hormonal Chaos,* calculated that even if just the most common one thousand chemicals were tested in unique combinations of three at a single dose per experiment, it would take 166 million different experiments to cover all of the possibilities. With up to one hundred thousand separate synthetic chemicals in production and in the marketplace, the potential number of synergistic combinations becomes mind-boggling. Krimsky estimates it could take "over a thousand years" to complete a chemical-by-chemical testing program, "an effort that would involve a level of complexity that could easily overwhelm our most advanced testing systems and surely our federal budget."

THERE IS TRUTH IN LABELING

Snake oil salesmen used to peddle their wares from town to town during the nineteenth century, touting the "special secret ingredients" in their tonics as cure-alls for most every ailment afflicting humankind. Today we find the modern equivalent within the chemical, drug, and food industries, each of which uses trade secrecy laws designed to protect ingredients from imitation by competitors as a way to hide their special chemical ingredients from public view.

From the manufacturer's perspective the trade secrets help to protect their patented ingredients from competitors, but in practical terms most competitors are sophisticated and wealthy enough to use reverse engineering in the laboratory to identify the ingredients of most any product on the market. The biggest net effect of trade secrecy is to deny the public an opportunity to assess the complete picture of chemical risks and safety for the products they purchase. Even if all ingredients were clearly listed, how could consumers be expected to know what is safe and what is potentially harmful?

The only "truth" in labeling today is the fact that there is widespread secrecy. Of forty common consumer products tested by the National Environmental Trust in Washington, D.C., during 2004, more than half contained toxic chemicals not listed on the product labels. Two examples cited were Lysol All Purpose Cleaner, containing unlisted glycol ethers (a neurotoxin), and Revlon Moondrops Lipsticks, containing unlabeled phthalates that are neurotoxins and reproductive toxins. Food additives may be labeled simply "flavorings" or "natural," while chemicals in personal-care products might fall under "fragrances" or "unscented," and pesticide ingredients hide under the term "inert." Genetically modified foods aren't labeled either, though we can be sure the GMOs (Genetically Modified Organisms) are now in just about every processed food product we encounter.

Let's break down these terms to see what they really mean. Fragrances are chemicals used to either add a pleasing aroma to cosmetics or other products, or to mask a hideous odor from other chemicals in the product. Even products labeled "unscented" or "fragrance-free" may contain these masking ingredients. This practice certainly sounds deceptive to me, as does the tendency of food processors to hide synthetic chemicals under the "natural flavors" language. "The individual components that make up the fragrance portion do not have to be listed on the label," according to a 2002 issue of *Flavour and Fragrance Journal,* a chemical science publication. "Only the word 'fragrance' must appear. The fragrance portion of the product may contain over one hundred different materials. . . . Secrecy is often required to protect the formula."

While pesticides containing fragrances must have their chemical mixtures registered with the United States Environmental Protection Agency, the EPA is prevented by law from revealing these fragrance ingredients to the public because it is deemed to be confidential business information. In 1999 this secrecy proved detrimental to the public health. Two products designed to kill dust mites entered the marketplace and quickly generated hundreds of health complaints from consumers. It turned out the "fragrances" in these products were responsible. Though the EPA recalled the products from distribution in 2000, it never revealed exactly which chemicals produced the health problems.

Another level of secrecy surrounding pesticide information concerns how the same ingredient can be labeled "active" in one product, making it subject to identification, then labeled "inert" in another product to render it a trade secret. Inert means the chemical doesn't have a direct killing effect on pests. Usually these ingredients are added to help the pesticide to dissolve in water, make it easier to apply, stabilize the product for longer shelf life, or to help the pesticide penetrate the insects' bodies.

A Canadian physicist, Dr. John Sankey, became curious about the real meaning of "inert" and examined data about pesticides collected by the Canadian government. He discovered eight thousand pesticide formulations registered for use in that country, containing about five hundred "active" ingredients, but there were at least another one thousand chemical ingredients in the products categorized as "inert," meaning they didn't have to be identified on product labels.

The term "inert" is absurd, Sankey concluded, "because no company is going to pay good money to put something into a pesticide product that doesn't do anything! Let alone spend millions on lawyers to protect the identity of those substances as trade secrets! It is unacceptable science to deliberately use a word to classify something in a way that is the direct opposite of what that word means."

In the United States, up to 99 percent of ingredients in any product can be withheld from labels under trade secrecy laws if they are categorized as "inert" or "other," which amounts to at least 2,500 substances added secretly to products. Most inerts are in bug sprays, insect repellents, and other pesticide products. Toxins expert Doris J. Rapp claims that at least two hundred chemicals classified as "inert" are environmental pollutants hazardous to human health, while a group called the Northwest Coalition for Alternatives to Pesticides puts the number of hazardous "inert" chemicals at 650 or more.

Rapp identifies five so-called inerts in a single herbicide, triclopyr, and each of those five chemicals has been linked in laboratory studies to tumors, elevated blood pressure, respiratory illness, kidney damage, and vision loss. Other cancer-causing chemicals classified as "inerts" include benzene, a solvent used in plastics and textiles; xylene, used in plastics and inks; and cristobalite, an "inert" known to be carcinogenic and used in over 1,500 pesticide products. An "inert" ingredient called POEA, which is added to the herbicide Roundup, has been shown in laboratory experiments to kill frogs and other amphibians.

A classic case of an "inert" ingredient causing health problems in humans is vinyl chloride, used as a propellant in such aerosol products as deodorants and hair sprays. Not until an epidemic of cancers began turning up in chemical plant workers who made vinyl chloride did the manufacturers realize this "inert" was a killer. Back then, in 1973, vinyl chloride was being used by every hairdresser in the nation. A PBS documentary eventually revealed, according to the PBS Web site, how "rather than warn beauty parlor operators, or urge that the hair spray be recalled, the manufacturers decided to quietly get out of the aerosol business" in an attempt to avoid liability lawsuits. "It is impossible to know how many women may have been sick or died—without knowing why."

MYTHS WE CHERISH

THE POISON IS IN THE DOSE

We are told by mainstream science, medicine, and industry that we shouldn't be concerned about our toxic body burden because "the poison is in the dose," a mantra that is the foundation for our public health standards. We are reminded that too much of just about anything can cause health problems, an idea originally advanced by a Swiss physician, Paracelsus, known as the father of toxicology, who in the sixteenth century wrote that "the right dose differentiates a poison from a remedy."

By this standard as well as in practice, vitamin A is good for us, but too much vitamin A causes liver damage. Vitamin D is good for us, but too much of it harms the kidneys. Similarly, eating spinach can be nutritionally good for us, but if we were to eat fifteen pounds of it at a single sitting, we might suffer permanent kidney damage from the oxalic acid that occurs naturally in spinach.

But does this fundamental premise of modern toxicology remain true when it comes to designer chemicals taking up residence in the human body? Based on emerging evidence, it is safe to say the answer is no. New chemicals and new mixtures of chemicals that have never entered the human body before are being absorbed. These are substances that break down very slowly in the body and are sometimes even indestructible. They don't follow the old public health rules of what is known to be risky.

Many synthetic chemicals are biologically active at incredibly low levels. Effects are occurring in the human body even when the dose seems far below what is usually considered a threshold. With PCBs it only takes five parts per billion in a mother's blood—the equivalent of one drop of water in 118 bathtubs of water—to cause permanent brain damage to a fetus in the womb. Studies done at the University of Missouri have found that very low levels—two parts per billion—of bisphenol A, a chemical found in plastics, disrupts the endocrine systems of laboratory animals, causing birth defects. By way of analogy, two parts per billion is comparable to two sheets in a roll of toilet paper stretching from New York to London.

MYTHS WE CHERISH

WE CAN HANDLE THE BODY BURDEN

Mainstream physicians and toxicologists assure us that a frontline defense of healthy livers and kidneys will keep us safe from nearly all levels of toxic accumulation. "Most Americans have hundreds of toxins stored in their livers, and the liver is very capable of taking this kind of chemical load," says James Dillard, assistant clinical professor of Columbia University's College of Physicians & Surgeons, whose comment typifies this point of view.

There can be no doubt the human liver constitutes a wondrous and magnificent organ. Whether toxins enter our bodies through skin, lungs, or stomach, these intruders must eventually confront the liver, where they are detected and then usually dispatched in one of three ways: being locked away into the far reaches of the liver itself, sent on for elimination in the filtering system of the kidneys, or stored away in fat cells.

It is in these fat cells that many of the long-term problems arise. Chemicals that persist in the body because they cannot be rapidly broken down or excreted create what is referred to in biomonitoring as the body burden. A growing chorus of medical experts insists that the inability of our bodies to excrete these toxins in a timely manner is in itself a cause for concern because our physical systems were never meant to metabolize the exotic range of synthetics we encounter.

"Unfortunately our bodies were never designed to protect themselves against this chemical onslaught," observes Paula Baillie-Hamilton, a British authority on the health effects of toxic chemicals. "As a result, our systems usually fail to process and remove most of these chemicals once they have entered our bodies, so their levels start building up inside us. Consequently, every single human on the face of this earth is now permanently contaminated with these modern synthetic chemicals."

Consider how a single toxin appearing in a widely used product called Scotchgard ended up accumulating in the body tissues of just about every human being on the planet and created a huge health scare that continues to this day. Scotchgard is produced by the 3M Company as a stain-resistant coating for fabrics, leather, furniture, and carpets, and its active ingredient perfluorooctane sulfonic acid (PFOS) even found its way into the packaging of processed foods and fast foods. PFOS residues began turning up in the blood of the general population and in wildlife as early as 1976, and in 1983 a long-term study of PFOS in rats found that it stimulated the growth of cancerous liver tumors. Yet, inexplicably this product remained on the market.

By the time the Centers for Disease Control and Prevention began biomonitoring in 1999, the PFOS chemical had been detected in the blood of most people everywhere from the United States to Sweden. Tests indicated that it persisted in human tissues for up to four years and had "bioaccumulation and toxicity properties to an extraordinary degree," according to the EPA.

Finally, in May 2000, under pressure from the EPA, these PFOS chemicals were phased out of 3M products, but they persist in our blood and fat cells and in our surrounding environment. When it comes to excretion, our livers are defenseless against this toxin and hundreds more like it.

Candor about the persistent body burden of chemicals we all bear comes from the British government's Health Protection Agency, which issued this public admission in 2005: "The long-term consequences of low-level, chronic exposure to chemicals and poisons are not well understood." A study done for the American Institute of Biological Sciences made a similar observation: "concern has grown about chronic effects of long-term exposure to relatively low doses of contaminants. . . . small daily doses of some contaminants will create cumulative effects that eventually impair our health. . . ."

An important factor rarely considered by apologists for the synthetics belief system is how single chemicals that seem benign by themselves can become monsters when they interact as an additive effect or synergistically with other chemicals to greatly magnify their effects. You will find more about the hidden role of synergies in chapter two.

PLAYING BIOLOGICAL ROULETTE

Mixing synthetic chemicals in our bodies has become tantamount to playing with a chemistry set without an instruction manual. During a speech before the 1994 conference of the American College for the Advancement of Medicine, an internationally recognized expert in toxicology, Samuel Epstein, predicted that one-third of us will get cancer in our lifetimes as a result of this chemical experiment. A decade later other cancer researchers increased the odds to one out of every two of us being diagnosed with cancer at some point in our lives.

A cancer study compiled in 2005 by three medical science researchers at the University of Massachusetts provided a half century of data showing the pattern of connections between synthetic chemical production and higher rates of cancer. From 1950 to 2001 the incidence for all types of cancer in the United States increased by 85 percent, and that was the age-adjusted rate, which means the increase has nothing to do with people living longer. The fastest-growing rate of cancer for any age group over the past two decades has been among children, who cannot be accused of having smoked or partied or worked or stressed themselves into a diseased state.

Since 1950, the year I was born, the explosive growth in certain types of cancer has become mind-numbing. Skin melanoma cases are up 690 percent. Prostate cancer up 286 percent. Thyroid cancer up 258 percent. Non-Hodgkin's lymphoma up 249 percent. Liver and intrahepatic cancer up 234 percent. Kidney and renal pelvis cancers up 182 percent, and the list goes on. What triggered this huge explosion in cases of cancer?

In his speech Dr. Epstein laid the blame squarely on the synthetics chemical revolution. He described how in 1940, by using new technology, synthetic chemicals were created that had never existed before. With the advent of thermal and catalytic cracking, it became possible to take petroleum and isolate particular chemicals and then, with a process of molecular splicing and recombination to produce any chemical you wanted to produce.

"In 1940, we produced about one billion pounds of new synthetic chemicals. By 1950, the figure had reached fifty billion pounds, and by the late 1980s, it became 500 billion pounds, including a wide range of toxic, carcinogenic, neurotoxic and other chemicals. Most of these chemicals have never been tested for toxic, carcinogenic or environmental effects."

The National Institute of Environmental Health Sciences, a branch of the federal government's National Institutes of Health, has posted a fact sheet on its Web site that makes a rather remarkable admission. It is a direct challenge to the synthetic belief system's assurances that having these chemicals in our bodies and in the environment is normal and a benign additive to nature, and to our own nature:

"We're struggling to look at where genetics and the environment interact in the human cell, causing a molecule to change that starts a kind of chain reaction leading to disease. Scientists liken the changes to a cascade—a series of ever-larger waterfalls of cellular changes—that may lead to cancer, Parkinson's, arthritis, heart disease or other diseases. Though we still do not understand the root causes of many of these serious chronic diseases, we suspect they can be caused or triggered by chemicals and other environmental exposures from years before."

Within the collection of essays that form the book *Ecological Medicine*, published in 2004, is this forthright and brilliant summary by Kenny Ausubel of the dilemma that challenges all of us: "For decades, the scientific and medical community has accepted that a certain amount of pollution and disease is just the price we have to pay for modern life. This is called the 'risk paradigm,' and it essentially means that it is society's burden to prove that new technologies and industrial processes are harmful, usually one chemical or technology at a time. The risk paradigm assumes that there are 'acceptable' levels of contamination the earth and our bodies can assimilate. It also allows a small, self-interested elite to set these levels, undistracted by the 'irrational' fears and demands of the public. The 'science' behind it is driven by large commercial interests and can hardly be considered impartial or in the public interest. Viewed with any distance at all, the risk paradigm is at best a high-stakes game of biological roulette with all the chambers loaded."

We are confronted every day of our lives by chemical toxins with the potential to harm us. It seems as if there is no escape. So let's be honest

with each other. By willingly participating in the risky synthetics paradigm we have implicitly agreed to a social contract in which we are
each playing the role of guinea pig in a continuing chemical and genetic
experiment.

Some of us will sicken or die during this experiment. A few of us might
mutate and evolve effective immune system defenses. Others of us will decide to no longer play this deadly game. Once the genie of awareness is set
loose, once denial is penetrated and the truth is spoken, none of us have
an excuse to play the innocent victim anymore.

CHAPTER TWO

FROM THE WOMB TO THE GRAVE

"Chemicals have replaced bacteria and viruses as the main threat to human health. . . . The diseases we're beginning to see as the major causes of death in the latter part of this century and into the 21st century are diseases of chemical origin."

—Rick Irvin, a toxicologist at Texas A&M University

Southwest of Reykjavik, the capital of Iceland, you will find a small town that bases its economy on tourists coming to be in the presence of invisible beings called elves, gnomes, and fairies, the "hidden people." Clairvoyants created maps of these invisible realms, and earnest town leaders sell tourists the maps showing where the invisible beings live in villages. The tourists are told to be careful where they walk because, even though the invisible beings live at a different frequency than humans, our presence can still create disruptions in their world, a relationship that also presumably works in reverse.

By way of analogy to the synthetics paradigm, the leaders of our chemical, food, and drug industries assure us that within the invisible realm of molecules exists a benign but synthetic world that they have created and they control, and if we just follow the maps they sell us and watch where we step, we will experience the magic. We are told that as long as we trust the mapmakers and believe in their promise of a better life through their chemical "magic bullets" in our foods, medicines, and consumer products, our lives won't be disrupted, and we'll be safe from harm.

While this isn't a scam being consciously perpetuated by the industry leaders, we are still acting out a sort of mythology that impacts our health and our survival as a species. An entire economy has been built on the existence of an invisible realm, and we have become its tourists. There are some secrets about this invisible realm that may help to free you from its illusions.

THE HIDDEN ROLE OF SYNERGIES

For some unknown reason residents of the small oceanside town of Brick, New Jersey, population 76,119, began seeing alarming numbers of autism cases among its children in the late 1990s. This neurological disorder, which inhibits a child's communication and social interaction skills, was afflicting children in Brick at a rate three times the national average. A group of parents of autistic children, led by William and Bobbie Gallagher, suspected the reason might be a mix of three synthetic chemical contaminants in wells supplying Brick's municipal water.

The levels of each contaminant measured individually seemed too low to pose a threat to health. But common sense and intuition led these parents to propose that a synergy of the three primary water contaminants might account for the upsurge in autism. "What no one ever looks at is the cumulative effect of these chemicals," Bobbie, the mother of two autistic children, informed other parents. "That's one of the scariest things about when they do these studies. They only look at each compound individually."

These comments in news stories attracted the attention of three scientists at the Marine Biological Laboratory at Woods Hole, Massachusetts. They decided to conduct an experiment using the same combination of contaminants present in Brick's water supply and test it on the nervous system development of shellfish embryos. The study and its results, published in a 2005 issue of the peer-reviewed scientific journal *Environmental Toxicology and Pharmacology*, became a milestone in research linking synthetic chemicals and disease.

When the researchers treated the shellfish embryos, which are a useful model for studying cell development, with a cocktail of the three contaminants, an enzyme believed to be involved in neural development was significantly boosted. If that had occurred in human fetuses as a result of exposure to these contaminants—which may have happened from the mothers drinking chemical-laced water or bathing in it—then neural development could have been affected and autism might have resulted.

The implications of this study threaten to shake the synthetics paradigm to its core. Synergy means the simultaneous action of two or more chemicals (or processes) in which the total effect is much greater than the sum of their individual effects. What makes synergy so scary for scientists and government regulators—and even more so for corporate executives—is how it profoundly challenges all traditional risk analysis calculations of whether chemicals in products, food, water, or medicines pose a threat to human health.

Measurement techniques used by science and medicine remain too cumbersome to even begin projecting the risks of multiple chemicals from multiple sources interacting inside the human body. Many scientists and most corporations would rather pretend that synergies don't exist rather than face the prospect of having to admit that everything they thought they knew about synthetics and health is wrong.

A vast and largely uncharted research territory for science and medicine is the role of synergy in determining the quality of our health. Synergy "is actually one of the great governing principles of the natural world," contends biologist Peter Corning, author of *Nature's Magic*. He argues that synergy "ranks up there with such heavyweight concepts as gravity, entropy, and information" as a key to understanding how the world works.

Synergies influence our lives in multiple ways—for better and for worse. The human mind is a synergy of chemical reactions. So is human reproduction. So is our body's metabolizing of food. Even though *synergos*, a Greek word for "working together," implies cooperative effects that are positive, we do experience negative synergies, sometimes referred to as *dysergies*. The most obvious are prescription drug interactions that produce toxic side effects, such as when tranquilizers combine with pain-killers to cause coma or death.

Despite their central role in our lives, synergistic effects in the human body remain a mystery largely unstudied by medical science. "Scientists study complex systems through the lenses of their own specialized concepts, paradigms, and theories," writes Corning. "To many scientists, in fact, synergy is an unfamiliar term." We can underscore Corning's observation with this disturbing admission from 2004 by the editors of *Environmental Science & Technology*, an American Chemical Society journal: "It is a virtual certainty that other [chemical synergy] effects are occurring in the field that we are presently overlooking in the lab. How can all bio-diversity be protected from the myriad of chemicals they are now exposed to when . . . we do not even know what is there?"

One of the first references in mainstream literature to the potential impact of synergies came in the book *Silent Spring*, the 1962 environmental-themed bestseller by Rachel Carson, in which she sounded an alarm about the toxic effects on health of "two or more different carcinogens acting together." She cited two examples. When a phosphate pesticide called malathion is administered simultaneously with other phosphates, "a massive poisoning results—up to fifty times as severe as would be predicted on the basis of adding together the toxicities of the two." Similarly, when DDT is added to "other liver-damaging hydrocarbons, which are so widely used as solvents, paint removers, degreasing agents, dry-cleaning fluids," one chemical acts on another to alter and intensify its effect, a process that can produce cancer in humans.

In the early 1970s more evidence of toxic synergies emerged from the research work of Samuel Epstein at the Children's Cancer Research Foundation in Boston, and Keiji Fujii of Tokyo's National Institute of Hygienic Sciences. They discovered how two or more chemicals in combination could increase the overall toxic effects even when there was a separation of up to two hundred days between one chemical being added to another.

A broad spectrum of more recent evidence points to a myriad of ways in which synthetic chemical synergies may be having an impact on our health. The following examples illustrate how some of us are canaries in a coal mine, alerting the rest of us to an accumulating danger.

- A two-year University of Liverpool (England) laboratory study of four common food additives—the artificial sweetener aspartame, monosodium glutamate (MSG), and the artificial colorings quinoline yellow and brilliant blue—found them to interact synergistically in ways that interfere with the normal development of nerve cells. The mixtures of the additives had up to seven times greater neurotoxic effects on nerve cell growth when combined than when the additives were applied individually, concluded the December 2005 study in the journal *Toxicological Sciences*. The combinations of additives studied were typically what are found in a child's bloodstream after a snack and drink.
- A chemist at the Massachusetts Institute of Technology, Dr. Gerald Wogan, studied a group of men in Shanghai, China, and was "astonished" to discover that the risk of liver cancer in these men increased seventy times if they ingested chemical toxins from their food while infected with hepatitis B. The cancer-causing agents "were amplifying each other's effects," observed *The New York Times* (Dec. 13, 2005). "Further complicating the issue is that a person's diet, or components of the diet, can increase the activity of enzymes that convert chemicals into carcinogens. And other dietary components can inactivate enzymes that detoxify chemicals."
- Discussing the latest research on how long-term exposure to toxic chemicals destroys brain neurons and triggers Parkinson's disease, an epidemiologist with the National Institute of Environmental Health Sciences told the *Los Angeles Times* (Nov. 27, 2005): "It's not one nasty thing that is causing Parkinson's. It's exposure to a combination of many environmental chemicals." Pesticides in various combinations are now considered a chief culprit as silent killers of braincells.
- Flight attendants for airlines throughout the world have been experiencing a range of health symptoms labeled *skypoxia*, char-

acterized by nausea, headaches, fatigue, slurred speech, memory lapses, and nervous tremors. Some toxicologists believe the symptoms are due to chemical fume synergies exacerbated by confined cabin spaces and jet fuel vapors. "The way fumes react synergistically with other chemicals may be at the bottom of the problem," says Professor Chris Winder at Australia's University of New South Wales. "Although very little is known about chemical synergy, the problem is very real because of the many ill flight attendants."

- Research by Canadian government scientists at Health Canada in 2001 discovered that when laboratory animals were exposed to tiny mixtures of several bug sprays and weed killers, mixtures known to contaminate humans, 80 percent of the babies were born dead and the rest showed abnormal behaviors. The death rate was unexpectedly high, the scientists reported, because each chemical in the mixture was applied in doses thought to be nonlethal. These synergistic effects may mean "our whole testing system for new pesticides may be too flawed to show their true dangers," confessed one of the scientists.

- After a half century and an estimated one million baby deaths worldwide, the mystery of sudden infant death syndrome has confounded pediatricians and health-care specialists. Now a chemist in New Zealand, Jim Sprott, makes a persuasive case that crib death is caused by toxic gases created by a synergy of chemicals, such as fire retardants, added to mattresses during their manufacture. A fungus that commonly grows in bedding may interact with the synthetic chemicals and heat, and create enough gas to asphyxiate babies, whose bodies are much more susceptible than children's or adults'. Since the late 1990s midwives and other health-care professionals have encouraged mothers to wrap baby mattresses in airtight protective coverings. Since this campaign began, the crib-death rate in New Zealand has fallen by 48 percent, according to health authorities.

- 100 percent of the 9,282 people who had their blood and urine tested by the Centers for Disease Control and Prevention were found to carry a toxic cocktail of thirteen pesticides on average. "While the government develops safety levels for each chemical separately, this study shows that in the real world we are exposed to multiple chemicals simultaneously," observed Margaret Reeves, senior scientist at the Pesticide Action Network. "The synergistic effects of multiple exposures are unknown, but a growing body of research suggests that even at very low levels, the combination of these chemicals can be harmful to our health."

- Chlorine is a chemical with the ability to transform other chemicals into mimics of estrogen, the female hormone. "Those who drink chlorinated water are at a higher risk of developing breast cancer," reports British toxins expert Paula Baillie-Hamilton. "It seems that chlorine reacts with some of the substances in the water to form trihalomethanes, compounds linked to breast cancer. This cancer-inducing effect has been demonstrated in a study performed on women drinking chlorinated tap water in Louisiana."

- Writing in *Environmental Health Perspectives*, a group of scientists in 1996 reported that mixtures of several PCBs with dioxin caused synergistic increases in toxicity eight hundred times above what had been predicted. ". . . biological synergy . . . may be more common than previously thought," the scientists concluded. "Furthermore, it is clear that environmental signals can produce synergistic biological responses."

Chemical synergies may provide an explanation for the many great mystery illnesses of the late twentieth century—chronic fatigue syndrome, Gulf War syndrome, irritable bowel syndrome, and multiple chemical sensitivity syndrome. In the case of Gulf War syndrome, researchers at Duke University Medical Center in Durham, North Carolina, mixed together two pesticide chemicals widely used by soldiers during the Gulf War with a drug soldiers had taken as a precaution against toxic gas-warfare agents. Test animals exposed to the synergy from these chemicals experienced neurological disorders similar to symptoms reported by Gulf War veterans.

Multiple chemical sensitivity is a term coined by an allergist, Theron

Randolph, who came to suspect in the 1980s that exposure to modern synthetic chemicals caused the many chronic symptoms he was encountering in patients, including migraines, nausea, vomiting, memory loss, joint pain, sinus congestion, and itchy eyes and throat. A National Academy of Sciences report estimates that 30 percent of the U.S. population now suffers from some symptoms of this syndrome, more than double the number of sufferers in a 1987 measurement.

Though no definitive test for diagnosis and no proven scientific mechanism has surfaced to explain multiple chemical sensitivity syndrome, the logic that Randolph used to support his theory of synergy sounds compelling. The human body is like a barrel filling up with small doses of many synthetic chemicals until it is full, and once that threshold is reached, any further chemical exposure sets in motion a series of allergic reactions. This analogy may also work in relation to the body burden of chemical toxins we all carry. There could be a tipping point of chemical exposure that triggers our genetic susceptibility to an illness or disease, or a tipping point that weakens our immune system and makes us vulnerable.

Government regulators aren't equipped, either with technological expertise or financial resources, to monitor, much less regulate, the occurrence of synergies resulting from our contact with chemicals in our products, food, water, air, or medicines. We must begin to do the self-monitoring and self-regulating on our own. Much of it will be trial and error based on common sense and intuition. Mistakes will inevitably be made. But sensitive observations of how we and others respond to contact with combinations of chemicals in daily life will reveal patterns that may help us to navigate the synergy minefield.

CLUES TO A HEALTH MYSTERY

Deep in the wine country north of San Francisco a friend of mine suffering from an advanced stage of Parkinson's disease offered me his insights. For months Solomon Vargas had attended the meetings of a support group for Parkinson's patients held at the Adventist Health hospital in

Saint Helena. These sessions were an opportunity for the thirty or so patients, all in their first or second stage of Parkinson's, to share experiences about how they coped with the physicial symptoms of tremors and spasms and the potent cocktail of drugs they were being given, drugs so toxic they needed to be monitored with regular blood tests.

Solomon had been a marriage, family, and child counselor until his Parkinson's tremors became so severe that, at forty-one years of age, he lost his driver's license and could no longer work. He was curious about his fellow patients and the triggers for the onset of their diseases, so he began taking informal surveys of their habits and lifestyles. They were a diverse group, the youngest twenty-five, the oldest fifty-five, almost equally divided between men and women. They had been employed as taxi drivers and waitresses and white-collar professionals. Two of his fellow patients were wealthy vineyard owners.

"There was only one common factor I found among the entire group of us," Solomon told me. "We all had grown up eating a bad diet. We all had been raised on processed foods, and once in adulthood, we had been hooked on fast food and junk food. We were deficient in proper nutrition for our entire lives, and then we came down with Parkinson's."

Mainstream medical science regards the causes of Parkinson's and related nerve degeneration diseases such as ALS—commonly known as Lou Gehrig's disease—as being largely unknown. A neurologist quoted in *The New York Times* during 2005 put it this way: ". . . about 10 percent of cases appear to be linked to genetic flaws, while the other 90 percent are a persistent mystery."

What we do know for certain is that neurodegenerative disorders have become an epidemic that increasingly strikes people before the age of forty, a stark contrast to less than two decades ago, when it was rare to find anyone under the age of sixty with these afflictions. One theory is that the disorders are triggered by exposure to mixtures of insecticides and other chemicals commonly used in agricultural areas such as the wine country of northern California, where my friend Solomon grew up.

After being diagnosed with the disease, Solomon did extensive research into brain and nerve functioning, and this information, combined with his surveys of fellow patients, led him to a commonsense revelation. "I have become convinced that a nutrient deficiency in our diets combines with all of the synthetic chemicals we are being exposed to, and this creates a toxic synergy with neurological disease effects."

I believe he is right—we weaken our immune systems with a diet of processed foods, then we expect our bodies to rally under an ever-increasing "body burden" of toxins.

In an attempt to get a grasp on the scope of synthetic chemicals that most of us are exposed to during the course of a "normal" life, along with the possible health effects of these chemicals acting individually or together, I sifted through the medical and scientific literature and compiled the following overview. It is by no means a complete or detailed picture of the hazards we face, but by dividing some of the more obvious exposures to toxins into five stages or phases of life, we get a sense of how and why our bodies have become so burdened with chemicals over a lifetime.

OUR FIVE TOXIC PHASES OF LIFE

Phase One: Fetal Development

For most of the twentieth century, medical science assured us that the placenta connecting a mother and a fetus acted as a foolproof filter, protecting the fetus from toxins absorbed by the mother's body during pregnancy. We now know this was a myth. You might remember how the first big public clue came in the 1980s with the "crack baby" epidemic. Children were being born addicted to crack cocaine, which their mothers had been using while pregnant. Suddenly, everything we thought we knew about fetal development and toxins became just another disproven and discarded theory.

Most chemical substances have been shown to be anywhere from three to ten times as toxic to fetuses and newborns as adults. This contamination can even begin at conception, as a result of the mother's body burden of chemicals, or the father's semen being a carrier for environmental toxins that can be introduced directly into the egg at fertilization. Here are a few of the chemical challenges every fetus must now contend with during its nine-month attempt to evolve into a normal being with naturally oc-curring health.

Air Pollution: If your mother lived in a big city, you were exposed to numerous types of air pollutants, pesticides from corner markets or rooftop gardens, and insecticides used in many apartment and commer-cial buildings. A 2005 study by Columbia University biologists found that prenatal exposure to pollutants was linked to genetic changes associ-ated with an increased risk of cancer in later life. A 50 percent increase in the level of persistent genetic abnormalities was found in infants whose mothers had high levels of pollution exposure in New York City. ". . . the simple act of an expectant mother breathing [polluted air] might cause chromosome abnormalities in the fetus," declared one biologist who co-authored the study.

Household Chemicals: After studying more than seven thousand chil-dren, a research team at the University of Bristol in Britain found in 2004 that children whose mothers made frequent use of chemical-based domes-tic products during pregnancy were more likely to develop asthma after birth. These products include disinfectants, bleach, aerosols, air freshen-ers, window cleaners, carpet cleaners, dry-cleaning fluids, and pesticides. A primary chemical culprit in most of these products seemed to be for-maldehyde. This study helps to explain why the incidence of childhood asthma has tripled in many industrialized countries since the 1970s.

Everyday Conveniences: Babies in the womb now swim in and absorb a synthetic chemical soup. While you were in the womb, there was about a one in three chance that you would absorb PCBs from your mother. (PCBs are toxins found in electrical transformers, hydraulic fluids, and adhesives.) PCBs have been detected in 30 percent of human breast milk, once again making your odds about one in three of having been exposed to additional PCB residue if you were breast-fed. PCBs at just five parts per billion in maternal blood during fetal development can cause adverse brain changes that can be permanent.

A 2004 study of ten randomly chosen babies born in the United States analyzed their umbilical cord blood and found an average of two hundred synthetic chemicals, including chemicals from food packaging, flame retardants from household furniture and appliances, and the Teflon chemical PFOA. Nearly every one of the chemicals has been linked to either cancer, brain and nervous system disorders, birth defects, or developmental problems.

Food Contamination: One of every six pregnancies involves exposure to methylmercury, at levels above EPA guidelines, from the consumption of mercury-laden seafood, primarily swordfish and canned white tuna, according to the Centers for Disease Control and Prevention. Mercury contamination of U.S. waterways is so widespread that forty states have issued health advisories for pregnant women or women of reproductive age. Mercury, along with PCBs and chlorinated pesticides, has been shown to disrupt the endocrine system, which manages hormones in the body.

An entire class of potential chemical contaminants to the fetus are the thousands of chemical additives in processed foods and fast foods. Observes Ross Hume Hall, a Canadian professor of biochemistry who is an expert on how synthetic chemicals damage human cells, "Chemical exposure during the fetal stage can set in motion tissue changes that years later, as an adult, erupt into cancer. None of the chemicals currently approved as food additives have ever been tested for their full potential to harm the unborn."

Phase Two: Childhood

Once out of the womb, you are confronted by a gauntlet of chemical challenges. By the time you are six months old you have already received 30 percent of your total lifetime toxic load of chemicals. Some kids start life with a genetic defect that affects metabolic functions and renders their bodies less efficient at excreting toxins. This predisposition can compromise their immune systems. The cocktail of vaccines that most children are injected with early in life, especially those vaccines containing the mercury-based preservative thimerosal, can further overwhelm the already susceptible child's immune system. From 1988 until 2002, when it was removed from most vaccines as a health threat, thimerosal was a primary source of toxic mercury exposure for most children, who received up to nine shots containing the additive by the time they were six months of age.

Food Additives: Because many of an infant's body organs are not fully developed at birth, infant growth can be retarded by contact with foreign chemicals. Organ cells in the infant are highly susceptible to chemical food additives, particularly the nitrites that sometimes appear in baby foods. Food additives in the form of synthetic colorings, flavorings, and preservatives, which lace all processed foods, increase your childhood chances of becoming hyperactive and developing attention deficit disorder. Numerous investigations have shown how, once foods containing synthetic color additives are removed from their diets, children exhibit much less hyperactivity. Behaviors connected to synthetic food additives include short attention span, restlessness, irritability, aggressiveness, and excitability. Even more than soft drinks, most fruit drinks (not fruit juices) are composed of synthetic chemicals that can trigger disruptive behaviors.

Breast Milk: Any baby born today or in the past decade who consumed its mother's breast milk also probably absorbed traces of perchlorate, a toxic component of rocket fuel. A 2005 study of lactating women in eighteen U.S. states found the toxin in practically every mother's milk. The source was food eaten by the mothers that had been tainted from irrigation water during the growing season. This water had been polluted by perchlorate seeping from defense industry plants scattered around the nation. A breast-fed one-month-old infant will absorb enough perchlorate to exceed all safe levels, perhaps even its lifetime safe level, as determined by a panel of the National Academy of Sciences. Perchlorate is known to adversely affect the thyroid (which controls your metabolism) and other glands of your body.

Infant Formula: For many, the first food you received after birth was infant formula, an artificial imitation milk. Many medical researchers point to infant formula as a primary cause of allergies in infants. Baby bodies were not designed to absorb synthetic chemicals. Mother's milk, by contrast, naturally contains colostrum, a substance that helps the infant develop protection against viral infections, influenza, dysentery, and a host of other diseases and ailments. Infant formula bestows no such protections.

Tap Water: If you drank fluoridated water as a child, depending on your consumption, your chances of contracting allergic reactions to the fluoride may increase with age, resulting in headaches, muscle weakness, and stomach upsets. At higher consumption levels, fluoride can cause retardation and other cognitive disabilities.

Childhood Vaccinations: If you grew up in the United States you had to receive a series of up to nine vaccinations for various diseases such as diphtheria before you could enter the public school system. These are mandatory vaccinations enforced by laws in each of the states. Many of these vaccines were administered to you as an infant. Numerous countries have similar requirements. Besides the disease-fighting agents, what else lurks in these vaccines that your body absorbed? "It's not the vaccines that are the problem—it's the additives," says Northeastern University pharmacy professor Richard Deth, a recognized expert on childhood vaccinations.

Common vaccine additives include methylmercury, aluminum, formaldehyde, MSG, sulfites, and ethylene glycol (which is also used as antifreeze). Most are used as preservatives and "adjuvants," a term referring to chemicals that can provoke your immune system into an early and longer-lasting response. Each of these additives, according to the British toxins authority Paula Baillie-Hamilton, has been linked to disorders ranging from brain and nerve damage to autism and attention deficit/hyperactivity disorder (ADHD). The overall amount of mercury that you as a child received from vaccinations may represent your entire lifetime's safe amount of mercury exposure. A 1999 United States Public Health Service warning confirmed that routine vaccinations are exposing many infants to quantities of mercury well above government health guidelines. "Ever since mass vaccination of infants began in the twentieth century, reports of serious brain, cardiovascular, metabolic and other injuries started filling pages of medical journals," says Baillie-Hamilton.

Household Dust: Though lead paints were banned throughout the United States in 1978, an estimated thirty-eight million homes still have this neurotoxin coating their walls, which may explain why one in six U.S. children tests as having high levels of lead in their blood. Lead lowers IQ, impairs memory, reduces attention spans, and causes learning disabilities. Molecules of lead leach from paint and attach themselves to dust particles that collect on furniture and on rugs and carpets, where crawling children inhale and absorb the particles. Pesticide and insecticide residues and chemicals that outgas from new carpeting also mix with dust, surviving in carpets and rugs for years until absorbed by humans or animals.

Play Areas: Pressure-treated wood used on outdoor decks, picnic tables, and playground equipment contains high levels of arsenic, according to the Environmental Working Group. A twelve-foot section of pressure-treated lumber contains about an ounce of arsenic, enough to poison to death 250 people. This wood is also injected with preservatives and toxins to prevent bug infestations. As children play on the surfaces of treated wood, the toxic chemicals can stick to their hands and then be ingested when they put their hands in their mouths. It is estimated that at least one out of every five hundred children who regularly play on playground equipment or decks will develop cancer later in life as a result of this exposure.

Food Packaging: Stain repellants that coat hundreds of products and are especially prevalent in food packaging leach a Teflon chemical known as PFOA into food, water, and the surrounding air. Blood testing has found the highest concentrations of this chemical in children six years of age and younger and in persons sixty years of age and older. Teflon molecules never break down in the environment and can persist in the human body for an entire lifetime.

The incidence of childhood brain and other central nervous system cancers rose by 26 percent between 1973 and 1996. Among girls born today, at least one in eight is expected to get breast cancer during her lifetime. If current trends continue, the granddaughters of today's young women will have a one-in-four chance of developing breast cancer.

"Children today live in a very different environment from years ago," says Philip Landrigan, a pediatrician who chairs the Department of Community and Preventative Medicine at the Mount Sinai Medical Center in New York. "There are new patterns of illness emerging and many more chemicals to which children are exposed. More than ten million products contain chemicals. Toxicity testing has not even begun to keep pace with disease. We are conducting a vast toxicological experiment on our children that will last for generations to come."

Phase Three: Teenage Years

Our internal cleansing systems, which naturally detoxify our bodies, were not designed to eliminate synthetic chemicals. As a result, many of the toxins bioaccumulate in our organs and tissues, and await a trigger to begin a synergistic process that can result in illness and disease. During our teen years, we experiment with an ever-wider range of chemicals in our bodies and on our bodies, from our first use of personal-care products to tattoo inks and illicit substances.

Processed Foods: If you are an average person, your teen years were spent acquiring food habits that would last a lifetime. Fast foods and processed foods, both categories laden with synthetic chemicals, bioaccumulated in your body from childhood and began to reach toxic levels during teenhood. Your mood swings that went beyond normal hormonal fluctuations became one observable symptom of this toxicity. If you became a hot-dog fanatic as a child or teenager and consumed a dozen or more each month, preservative chemicals found in the meat may have bioaccumulated and sharply elevated your risk of developing leukemia.

Fast Foods: Teenagers eat more french fries and fast food than any other age group. French fries have been consumed for generations, but only in

2005 did we discover that the act of frying starches creates a carcinogen. The obvious question is what else do we not know about the most common foods we eat?

Overprescribed Antibiotics: On average, every teenager in the United States receives at least one prescription for antibiotics every year. Most prescriptions are for sore throats, 90 percent of which are viral and not responsive to antibiotics. This unnecessary usage of antibiotics sets in motion a lifetime of unthinking use and exposures to deadly strains of resistent bacteria that prey upon immune systems weakened by the overuse of antibiotics.

Pesticide Exposure: Teenagers who have grown up in agricultural areas or in residential areas that adjoin crop-growing areas, such as Fresno, Sacramento, and other cities in the Central Valley of California, inherit a much higher body burden of chemical pesticides and herbicides. But everyone is at risk from pesticide residues on supermarket produce. Pesticide residues on nonorganic foods begin to accumulate in fatty tissues and organs at an early age. Studies of chemical body burdens done in the state of Washington found that children and teenagers who ate organic foods had significantly lower levels of pesticide contaminants in their bodies than kids who had a nonorganic diet.

Personal-Care Products: As a teenager you experiment with a wide array of personal-care products that include shampoos, aftershaves, deodorants, cosmetics, and antibacterial soaps. On average you will be exposed to two hundred new synthetic chemicals from these products. Some of the ingredients—called endocrine disrupters—affect hormone levels and lead to mood swings and other effects on behavior and mental acuity. The suntan oils and lotions you lather on your body during the summer contain at least seven chemicals that have been found to be carcinogens or endocrine disrupters.

Body Decorating: Many of you got your first tattoo when you were a teenager. Evidence has been emerging, most recently reported in *Medical*

News Today, that the synthetic dyes used in the inks needled into you were laced with heavy metals. These toxins can migrate through the body and lodge in various body organs, particularly the lungs.

Phase Four: Adulthood

Throughout your adult life you continue to accumulate synthetic chemical toxins in your body tissues, building on levels of exposure from the three earlier stages of life. Whether these exposures will trigger specific diseases and illnesses in you depends on a variety of factors, including your genetic predispositions and how badly your immune system has been battered by chemical toxins.

Meat Hormones: If you ate meat regularly between 1947 and 1977, especially beef, you were exposed to increasing levels of the sex hormone DES, which causes cancer. DES was administered to livestock to add weight and fat, and it remained an additive in the U.S. meat supply for three decades until it was removed as a health danger.

Food Additives: From 1948 on, most processed foods, including baby food, contained increasing levels of MSG as an additive. Lab tests find that animals given doses of MSG develop brain damage. Your use of diet drinks and 1,200 other food products containing the artificial sweetener aspartame has exposed you to the risk of 88 symptoms of toxicity, as identified by the U.S. Department of Health and Human Services. These range from allergies and headaches to more serious maladies affecting the nervous system.

Seafood Consumption: If you have been a regular consumer of seafood over the past three decades—two times or more a week—and it has primarily consisted of albacore white tuna in cans and swordfish, then your body burden of mercury contamination should be a cause for concern. Similarly, if you have regularly consumed fish caught in the Great Lakes, your absorption of PCBs has increased your chances of developing neurological impairments.

Cosmetics Use: If you are a woman and began using cosmetics as a teenager, you have absorbed a broad range of toxins, perhaps more than one thousand separate substances. The FDA estimates that about 65 percent of women's cosmetics contain potentially carcinogenic ingredients.

Pesticide Exposure: If you were born before 1974, you were exposed to the pesticide dieldrin, a dangerous carcinogen, which turned up in 96 percent of all meat and 85 percent of all dairy products tested in the United States. (Dieldrin was banned by the FDA in 1974.) If as a child you played on lawns or in gardens sprayed with the pesticide diazinon (banned in 2004), you were exposed to a toxin that is known to damage the nervous system.

Occupational Hazards: Researchers at the National Institute for Occupational Safety and Health studied more than 2.6 million U.S. death records and in 2005 reached these conclusions about brain degeneration health hazards associated with the type of job you choose: farmers exposed to pesticides and welders exposed to fumes from manganese have a higher than average incidence of Parkinson's disease; hairdressers are at a much higher risk for Alzheimer's and other motor neuron diseases because of their contact with hair dyes and solvents, as are aircraft mechanics from their exposures to toxic fuels and solvents; veterinarians and graders and sorters have the highest risk of dying from ALS, a wasting of the central nervous system.

Phase Five: Senior Years

By retirement the average person is taking at least one prescription drug a day to combat any one of dozens of common ailments. At this point in your life your total body load of chemicals has reached a critical threshold that makes you more susceptible to prostate cancer if you are a man and to breast cancer if you are a woman. A study released in late 2005 by the WWF, a conservation group in Switzerland, revealed blood-test results of children, mothers, and grandmothers in twelve European countries. The highest concentration of synthetic chemicals was in the oldest generation tested, providing the strongest evidence yet that chemicals bioaccumulate in the body over a lifetime. "It shows that we are all unwittingly the subjects of an uncontrolled global experiment," a WWF researcher told the Reuters news service.

Prescription Drugs: At least fifty-five commonly used medications—such as antibiotics and antihistamines—can create disorientation and weaken memory and cognitive abilities in the elderly. If you have abused antibiotics during the course of your life, taking them when they aren't needed, you have inadvertently made your immune system vulnerable to deadly strains of bacteria.

You have a one-in-four chance of taking three or more prescription drugs every day after retirement. Because your liver and kidney functions have diminished with age, the possible synergistic effects of these drugs increase your likelihood of an overdose and of becoming one of the one hundred thousand people who die in the United States each year from the synergies and side effects of prescription medications. Taking prescription drugs over extended periods also depletes your body of essential nutrients which, unless they are replaced with supplements, results in suppression of proper immune system functioning.

Tap Water Bioaccumulation: Throughout your years of life, the fluoride you have ingested and absorbed from municipal water supplies has bioaccumulated in your bones and made them more brittle. Your prospects for hip fractures during your senior years have been increased well beyond what you could have expected if you had drunk and bathed in only bottled water.

New Car Smells: By retirement age you have probably owned more than a few new cars in your life, and you may have enjoyed the unmistakable aroma of fresh upholstery, carpeting, plastic, and paint that a new vehicle exudes. Breathing in these fumes may have given you and your passengers a feeling of light-headedness, nausea, drowsiness, headaches, or a scratchy throat. That is because any chemical you can smell—whether it be vinyl in new shower curtains or vinyl in new cars—is making its way into your bloodstream when you inhale it. All these years you have been inhaling and absorbing a chemical brew of volatile organic compounds (VOCs), as they are called, composed of such cancer-causing chemicals as styrene and formaldehyde. These gases are even more dangerous on hot days when the windows are rolled up and the air conditioner is operating. Japanese carmakers have recognized this threat to health from toxic fumes and have agreed to reduce the cabin levels of thirteen VOCs to meet Japanese Ministry of Health, Labour and Welfare guidelines by 2007. In the United States and other Western countries, the air quality of new auto interiors has yet to become a priority for automakers.

Toxins expert Sherry A. Rogers actively disparages the idea, promoted by the chemical and food industries, that small amounts of toxins are harmless to the body. ". . . they neglect to mention that since we do not totally detoxify the everyday 'harmless' amounts of chemicals that we inhale and ingest, they silently stockpile [bioaccumulate] in our tissues. . . . studies are not routinely done on even the effects of one chemical decades later, much less the synergistic [exponentially damaging] effect of multiple chemicals. Decades later when they do cause disease, we still don't get the message. We chalk it up to old age."

YOUR PERSONAL TOXICITY TEST

Being toxic is an unavoidable consequence of living in the sea of synthetic chemicals that is our modern world. A healthy body is an efficient eliminator of toxins. We are aware of our daily elimination of feces and urine, two vital forms of elimination provided by our colon and kidneys, but there are other important forms of elimination. We have to breathe frequently and eliminate toxic carbon dioxide from our lungs. Our liver filters our blood supply of toxins. Our lymph system moves toxins and excess fluids from the body, as do our sweat glands. Our skin is also an elimination system. Any restriction or malfunctioning of these systems of elimination can cause toxins to accumulate, and illness or disease may result. We can tolerate a certain level of toxins in our bodies. For each person, this tolerance level will be different, depending on your exposure levels, your lifestyle, diet, drug intake, general habits, medical treatments, surrounding environment, the strength and clear functioning of your faculties of elimination, and the general strength of your immune system. Here is an opportunity to gauge your own level of toxicity.

Toxicity Questionnaire

INSTRUCTIONS
For each question, circle either YES or NO.

Select the one choice that most closely represents your individual situation. When you have finished answering all sixty-five questions, add up the number of circled YES answers.

1. Do you use plastic containers to store food or drinking water?

   YES   NO

2. Do you eat microwaved foods that come packaged with plastic wrap?

   YES   NO

3. Do you eat nonorganic cereals, bread, or other grain products?

   YES   NO

4. Do you use deodorants, shampoos, and soaps?

   YES   NO

5. Do you use aftershave, lotions, or perfumes?

   YES   NO

6. Do you use cosmetics or hair colorings?

   YES   NO

7. Do you live or work in an area that has synthetic carpeting?

   YES   NO

8. Do you live or work in an area that has wood cabinets or new furnishings?

YES   NO

9. Do you live or work near agricultural areas?

YES   NO

10. Do you live or work in an area that has painted walls or ceilings?

YES   NO

11. Do you drink nonorganic coffee?

YES   NO

12. Do you use sugar substitutes or eat any foods that contain low-calorie sugar substitutes or sweeteners?

YES   NO

13. Do you eat foods that contain hydrogenated fats, such as margarine, or do you eat any foods that contain canola oil or cottonseed oil?

YES   NO

14. Do you eat fat-free foods or snacks made with fat substitutes?

YES   NO

15. Do you ever drink tap water at home or at restaurants?

YES   NO

16. Do you eat nonorganic fruits, vegetables, grains, meats (all types), or dairy foods (all types)?

YES   NO

17. Do you breathe polluted air?

YES   NO

18. Do you drive a motor vehicle?

    YES   NO

19. Do you eat fish?

    YES   NO

20. Do you wear synthetic clothing or have your clothes dry-cleaned?

    YES   NO

21. Are you often irritable?

    YES   NO

22. Are you a smoker?

    YES   NO

23. Do you have difficulty breathing when anxious?

    YES   NO

24. Do you sometimes use bug-killers?

    YES   NO

25. Do you often have a loss of memory and inability to concentrate?

    YES   NO

26. Do you sometimes feel dizzy?

    YES   NO

27. Do you sometimes hear ringing or other sounds in your ears?

    YES   NO

28. Do you get skin rashes very easily?

    YES   NO

29. Do you have frequent urination in the night?

    YES   NO

30. Is your menstrual cycle often erratic or interrupted?

YES   NO

31. Do you have excessive hair loss?

YES   NO

32. Do you sometimes have unexplained numbness?

YES   NO

33. Do you often feel very fatigued or nauseous?

YES   NO

34. Does your speech sometimes become slurred or disordered?

YES   NO

35. Have you received three or more vaccinations?

YES   NO

36. Do you belong to one or more of the following groups, as a professional or hobbyist?
Agricultural product handlers, asbestos abatement technicians, auto mechanics, battery manufacturers, battery recyclers, canning plant workers, carpenters, ceramic manufacturers, construction workers, cooks, cosmetic manufacturers, cosmetologists, dental assistants, dental lab workers, dentists, diesel equipment mechanics, dynamite manufacturers, dynamiters, electronic assembly workers, electronic component manufacturers, electroplaters, engravers, explosives experts, farmers, fertilizer manufacturers, fiberglass installers, fiberglass manufacturers, firemen, firing range operators, fishermen, fluorescent tube manufacturers, food processors, foundry workers, glass manufacturers, glassblowers, grinder operators, hairdressers, hazardous material workers, ink manufacturers, jewelers, laboratory workers, landfill workers, landscapers, lumber processors, lumber yard workers, metal recyclers, metal sculptors, military soldiers, miners, nail technicians, painters (residental and commercial), paint manufacturers, pharmaceutical workers, photographers, physicians,

plastic product manufacturers, plumbers, plumbing supply manufacturers, policemen, potters, preservative manufacturers, printers, search-and-rescue workers, ship dock workers, smelting plant workers, solderers, tanners, tattoo artists, truck mechanics, waste handlers, well diggers

YES   NO

37. Do you have learning disabilities?

YES   NO

38. Do you have headaches?

YES   NO

39. Do you stutter or stammer?

YES   NO

40. Do you have chronic coughing?

YES   NO

41. Do you have heartburn?

YES   NO

42. Do you have mood swings?

YES   NO

43. Do you have depression?

YES   NO

44. Do you have hay fever?

YES   NO

45. Do you have insomnia?

YES   NO

46. Do you sometimes eat broiled, fried, or barbecued foods?

    YES   NO

47. Do you eat less than three servings of fruits and vegetables daily?

    YES   NO

48. Do you not eat whole-grain or natural-fiber foods daily?

    YES   NO

49. Do you rarely drink several glasses of pure water daily?

    YES   NO

50. Do you eat white flour foods and drink sodas often?

    YES   NO

51. Do you use home-cleaning products?

    YES   NO

52. Do you take synthetic vitamins daily or several times a week?

    YES   NO

53. Do you not exercise daily for thirty minutes or more?

    YES   NO

54. Are your bowel movements irregular?

    YES   NO

55. Do you travel in heavy commuter traffic daily?

    YES   NO

56. Do you eat fast food or frozen food at least twice a week?

    YES   NO

57. Does your family have a history of cancer, diabetes, heart disease, obesity, or depression?

YES   NO

58. Have you had cancer, diabetes, heart disease, depression, obesity, liver disease, or high blood pressure?

YES   NO

59. Do you have metal fillings in your teeth, and have you had dental surgery?

YES   NO

60. Are you under significant daily stress?

YES   NO

61. Do you use prescription drugs or illegal nonprescription drugs?

YES   NO

62. Have you had surgery that used anesthesia?

YES   NO

63. Do you have temporal mandibular joint issues?

YES   NO

64. Do you often feel bloated?

YES   NO

65. Have you had suicidal thoughts?

YES   NO

Number of YES answers _____

Your total number of YES answers determines your relative toxicity level. (Please note: This is not a scientific test or health evaluation. It simply suggests the possible extent to which you carry a body burden of chemicals.)

1-15   Mildly Toxic
16-28   Generally Toxic
29-45   Very Toxic
46-65   Severely Toxic

As you no doubt noticed, you are toxic even if you answered only a few questions in the affirmative. Toxicity varies only by degree. That reality generally reflects the findings from widespread blood tests conducted by the U.S. Centers for Disease Control and Prevention. Now let's explore the hows and whys of what brought us to this unavoidable state of contamination.

CHAPTER THREE

A HISTORY OF THE HUNDRED-YEAR LIE

An appropriate date to mark the beginning of the Hundred-Year Lie would be 1906, the year the U.S. Congress enacted the Pure Food and Drug Act, a law that for the first time gave Americans the illusion of food and drug safety and provided a legal standard for most other governments of the world to follow. Prior to its passage in early 1906, the chief chemist of the U.S. Bureau of Chemistry, Harvey Wiley, had urged the Congress to control drugs and food sold in interstate commerce because "I have found that the foods we daily consume are so fraught with germ life of a harmful nature that I am almost afraid to go to the table." Germs were identified as Public Enemy Number One, and synthetic chemicals in food and medicine were hailed as the cure for this germ threat.

Perhaps more than any other people on the planet, we North Americans have embraced the theme of "better living through chemistry." Its origins as an actual slogan go back to the aftermath of World War I, a conflict during which chemical companies profited handsomely from the manufacture of poison gas and other munitions. Executives at the DuPont Company, reacting to having been labeled "merchants of death," hired public relations advisers and even psychologists to shape a marketing campaign to rehabilitate the chemical industry's image. One result was an advertising slogan, "Better Things for Better Living . . . Through Chemistry." Decades later it was the Monsanto Company that took this theme of synthetics being natural to new heights of hyperbole with this statement touting its genetically modified foods: ". . . there really isn't much difference between foods made by Mother Nature and those made by man. What's artificial is the line drawn between them."

Our diets and our health, from the womb to the grave, are now shaped by three sectors of the economy: the processed foods corporations, the medical/pharmaceutical giants, and the chemical industry. Together these economic interests have fostered a belief system—a belief that most of us have naively embraced—promoting synthetics as benign and superior to naturally occurring foods and medicines. Blinded by ambition and the spirit of progress and commerce, we have unwittingly created an unstoppable force. The following factual chronology of the changes we have seen in the last one hundred years documents the slippery slope of discoveries, industrial developments, government actions, and accumulating health problems. Read this chronology straight through, and the patterns that constitute the Hundred-Year Lie will emerge.

The Slippery Slope Index

STAGE ONE: 1900–1939

A SYNTHETICS BELIEF SYSTEM EMERGES

At the outset of the twentieth century our food supply became an initial testing ground for innovations in the emerging "better living through chemistry" belief system. Chemists work with food processing companies to create artificial sweeteners, a butter substitute, taste-enhancing additives such as MSG, and the first partially hydrogenated vegetable shortening. These synthetics set the stage for the revolution in food processing that is to come.

1900   **Cancer** is the tenth leading cause of death in the United States, responsible for only **three percent of all deaths**. By the end of the twentieth century, cancer will be the cause of **20 percent of all deaths** in the United States.

   Diabetes affects less than one-tenth of one percent of the U.S. population; by the end of the twentieth century, **almost 20 percent** of U.S. citizens will contract type 1 or type 2 diabetes.

   Asthma and related immune system diseases are virtually

nonexistent; by the end of the twentieth century at least 150 million people worldwide will be afflicted.

Breast cancer in women is very rare; by 1960, breast cancer will affect one in twenty women; by 2005, one in three women will develop breast cancer.

Led by the Heinz and Campbell companies, American **food processors**, with their preserved and canned foods, now account for 20 percent of the nation's manufacturing capacity.

Refined sugar replaces molasses in the average American diet. Sugar consumption will rise from over ten pounds per person per year, and by the end of the twentieth century it will be over 147 pounds per person per year. Studies will eventually find that the **process of refining sugar removes 90 percent of sugar cane components and, with them, the most valuable nutrients**, leaving only calories. Diets high in refined sugar will lead to diabetes, heart disease, gastric and duodenal ulcers, chronic infections, and tooth decay.

1901   The Monsanto Company is founded by a chemist to manufacture **saccharin**, the first artificial sweetener.

1902   In Saint Louis, twelve **children die** after taking a diphtheria **vaccine** contaminated with tetanus that had been administered by the city's own health department.

1906   The Pure Food and Drug Act is passed by Congress, enabling the federal government to remove a food or drug product from circulation if its proves unsafe. But food processors and drug manufacturers are **not required to prove their products are safe**; the burden is on government to prove the products are unsafe before they can be removed.

1908   A Japanese chemist identifies a chemical called **MSG** as responsible for the taste-enhancing properties of a seaweed known as kombu.

1909   German chemist Fritz Haber invents **chemical fertilizer** by breaking apart molecules of nitrogen gas in the presence of ammonia.

Procter & Gamble acquires the U.S. rights to a British patent on making **liquid vegetable oils solid** at room temperature.

1910   **Margarine, a chemical synthesization of vegetable oil**, is introduced as a substitute for butter; by 1950, the average American will consume eight pounds of margarine a year. This is the beginning of **highly saturated trans fats** entering the U.S. diet through processed foods, bringing with them higher **cholesterol** levels.

1911 The first **partially hydrogenated vegetable shortening**, Crisco, is introduced to the public.

Heart attacks as a result of coronary artery disease are almost unknown to physicians.

A new **grain-milling** process is discovered in which the germ and outer layers of the wheat grain are removed (thus unknowingly eliminating a source of **vitamins E and B**) and refined flour is created, allowing the manufacture of white bread.

1915 German chemist Fritz Haber invents a **chlorine gas chemical weapon** that is first used against French soldiers in trenches near the Belgian city of Ypres.

1920 From this date forward to 2000, U.S. production of **synthetic chemicals** will increase from less than one million pounds a year to more than **140 billion pounds a year**.

1921 General Mills Corporation creates a character named **Betty Crocker** to convince generations of Americans to use **processed foods**.

Prior to this date, a total of twenty reports of **endometriosis** in women has been reported worldwide; by the late 1990s, nearly 20 percent of all women of childbearing age in the United States are afflicted with endometriosis.

1923 Despite concerns about health hazards, tetraethyl **lead is added to gasoline** sold in the United States. Over the next few decades airborne lead will **toxify soil, water, and food**. The lead will lodge in human bones and cause prenatal damage to children's brains.

1929 PCBs are first manufactured for use in electrical transformers, hydraulic fluids, plasticizers, and adhesives. By 1977, studies will find that **PCBs bioaccumulate as a toxin** in body tissues; 94 percent of fish sampled nationwide will contain PCB residues; most women tested will show PCB residues in their breast milk.

An **additive used as a preservative in vaccines**, thimerosal (a form of mercury), is found to cause death in laboratory test subjects. Despite this finding, the additive will be used in most child-hood and other vaccines for the rest of the twentieth century.

1930   About three thousand people this year, out of a U.S. population of 123 million, will die of **heart disease**; by 1997, at least 727,000 people will die of heart disease out of a population of 248 million.

1931   In this year a girl named Virginia is born; she will become the old-est child diagnosed with the **new disease called autism**; her birth year is also the first year that **thimerosal** is used in vaccines.

1933   A workable method of synthesizing vitamin C is turned into a commercial success by the pharmaceutical company Roche.

  A muckraking book, *100 Million Guinea Pigs: Dangers in Everyday Foods, Drugs, and Cosmetics,* is published and becomes a bestseller. It reveals **many cases of harm and death** from such products as eyelash liners that blind women, hair removal creams made from rat poison, and a weight-loss drug that causes cataracts.

  An *American Journal of Medicine* paper identifies a **new type of diabetes resistant to insulin,** called type 2 diabetes, which is be-coming an epidemic in the United States.

1935   Only one case of **cancer** has been reported among the Inuit of Alaska and Canada in the previous fifty years; from this date for-ward into the 1970s, after the Inuit adopt a **processed-foods diet,** their cancer rate will explode until it rivals other U.S. and Cana-dian consumers.

1936   A report published by a committee of the U.S. Senate warns the American public: "Do you know that most of us today are suffer-ing from certain dangerous **diet deficiencies which cannot be remedied until the depleted soils from which our foods come are brought into proper mineral balance?**"

1937   A Danish scientist publishes a book, *Fluorine Intoxication,* describ-ing hundreds of scientific studies indicating that **fluoride poisons** human and animal life, and especially affects the central nervous system.

1938   Pharmaceutical maker Roche, having mastered the industrial syn-thesis of vitamins A, B_1, B_2, E, and K, becomes the world's leading supplier of vitamins.

  A new federal law, the Food, Drug and Cosmetics Act, takes effect. Though the law empowers the Food and Drug Administration to force manufacturers to **prove their products are safe** before marketing them, the FDA chooses to focus enforcement efforts on the accuracy of information on product labels.

A powerful new pesticide called **DDT** is discovered by a Swiss chemist; in this same year British scientists synthesize a **synthetic estrogen** called **DES.**

From this date until 1990, average human **male sperm counts** will drop by almost 50 percent; during the same period the incidence of **testicular cancer** will triple.

1939   The first proposal to add **fluoride** to public water supplies is made by a scientist working under a grant from the Aluminum Company of America.

STAGE TWO: 1940–1961

SYNTHETICS TRANFORM LIFESTYLES

Our lives are fundamentally altered by a series of synthetic chemical discoveries made in the years before and after World War II. The pharmaceutical, pesticide, and fluoridation industries sink deep economic roots during this period, and synthetics in food, clothing, and household products become widely accepted as necessities of convenience.

1940   The **petrochemical era is born.** Using new technology that involves thermal and catalytic cracking, synthetic chemicals that have never existed before are created from petroleum. From this date forward to 1982, the production of synthetic chemicals increases 350 times; a new chemical substance is being discovered every nine seconds of every workday.

1941   The FDA approves **DES** for use as a treatment for **menopausal women.** Later the FDA will extend DES use to a variety of conditions associated with pregnancy.

1942   Physicians for the first time find a strain of bacteria—staphylococci—that has developed a **resistance to penicillin**; within a decade this strain will appear regularly in hospitals.

1945   America's **fluoridation** of its water supplies begins when 107 barrels of sodium fluoride are added to the Grand Rapids, Michigan, water supply.

    Nerve gas research conducted during the war results in the development of **chemicals toxic to insects**, producing an explosion in the production of pesticides.

1946   Strains of gonorrhea **resistent to penicillin** emerge.

    A trend of widespread patenting of individual drugs and their chemical ingredients by U.S. pharmaceutical companies begins; previously the attitude of these drug companies has been to avoid patenting them, in order to remain ethical in the eyes of consumers. Now drug manufacturers can keep drug prices artificially high.

1947   **Sex hormones** are first introduced into **livestock** production to add more fat and weight on the animals. One of those hormones, DES, is hailed as the most important development in the history of food production. Several decades later **DES will be found to cause cancer**. Even after the FDA bans this substance, cattle will continue to be administered illegal doses of DES.

1948   From this date forward the American food industry will double its use of **MSG** every decade, adding it to **processed foods**, including **baby food**. By the end of the century, researchers will discover that MSG can trigger dozens of toxic reactions in the human body.

1949   The breast cancer rate for women is fifty-eight cases per one hundred thousand people; within forty years the breast cancer rate will be more than one hundred cases per one hundred thousand people. The lifetime risk of contracting **breast cancer will more than double**.

1950   Most of the nation's **cattle** spend their lives until slaughter grazing in open spaces, eating naturally occurring grasses; by the early 1970s, three-quarters of U.S. cattle will spend most of their lives in crowded feedlots, being **injected with antibiotics and hormones**, and being fed a diet that includes processed sewage, poultry litter, shredded newspaper, sawdust laced with ammonia, tallow, and grease.

From this date forward to 2000, the overall incidence of **cancer** in the United States **will rise by 55 percent**, with lung cancer due to smoking accounting for only one-quarter of this increase. Rates for breast cancer and colon cancer in males will increase during this period by 60 percent; testicular cancer by 100 percent; adult brain cancer by 80 percent; childhood cancer by 20 percent.

1951   The U.S. Congress passes a law that consumers must have prescriptions from physicians to purchase drugs that cannot be used safely without medical supervision.

1952   From this date forward to 1987, the production and use of **synthetic pesticides** in the United States will increase thirteen thousand times faster than before and just after World War II.

1953   George Waldbott, vice president of the American College of Allergists, issues a warning that even small amounts of **fluoride** in water can cause acute and **painful allergies**. Whenever Waldbott's own patients stop drinking fluoridated water, they no longer experience headaches, muscle weakness, and stomach upsets.

1956   Medical researcher Ancel Keys connects the consumption of **trans fats in partially hydrogenated vegetable oils to cardiovascular disease**.

Perfluorochemicals used in Teflon and other nonstick products are first introduced; by 2004, blood tests will reveal that **96 percent of U.S. children** have one of these nonbiodegradable chemicals in their bloodstreams.

1957   From this date until 1971, **paper companies will place PCBs** in their carbonless copy paper to enable typists to make multiple copies.

The Framingham Heart Study in Massachusetts reports that high cholesterol levels may increase the risk of **heart disease**.

1959   The Shell and Dow chemical companies produce DBCP for use as a **soil fumigant** to protect fruit crops; it is widely sprayed over vineyards and citrus orchards. Twenty years will go by before the EPA bans DBCP as a dangerous toxin. Hundreds if not thousands of **men will become sterile** from contact with the fumigant.

1961   The FDA approves a medication called Ritalin for use by **children with behavior problems**. By 1975, about 150,000 children in the

United States will be taking Ritalin. By 2005, about six million U.S. children will be using Ritalin, representing 85 percent of total Ritalin consumption in the entire world.

STAGE THREE: 1962–1973

SYNTHETIC TOXINS MIGRATE

A watershed event in public policy comes in 1962 with the publication of Rachel Carson's book, Silent Spring, *which documents how toxic synthetic chemicals migrate through the environment and into the flesh of fish and other animals. The spread of toxic chemicals is not limited to pesticides, but as later studies will show includes a wide range of common synthetic chemicals that begin to contaminate all human bodies.*

1963 The drug thalidomide is given to pregnant women for morning sickness. More than six thousand babies will be born with **severe deformities** as a result of using the drug. Six years will go by before this drug is finally withdrawn from the marketplace.

1963 From this date forward, scholastic **aptitude scores** for U.S. high school children **plummet** every year. By the end of the century a possible link will be drawn to their consumption of food additives and other synthetic chemicals.

1964 From this date to 1992, **chemical pesticide use** in U.S. agriculture will increase by 300 percent, according to the USDA, though the total area of cropland under cultivation will remain virtually the same.

1965 A worldwide study of **heart disease** called the International Atherosclerotic Project studies twenty thousand autopsied human bodies from throughout the world and finds clear evidence that people who consumed more **saturated fats** had more heart attacks and more strokes.

A chemist working for G.D. Searle & Company discovers **aspartame**, an artificial sweetener.

1968 A scientist at Washington University in Saint Louis gives doses of

MSG to laboratory mice and discovers widespread **brain damage**, especially in immature and newborn animals.

A FDA report reveals that **lab animals fed irradiated foods** showed increases in pituitary cancer, testicular tumors, reduced fertility, and shortened life spans.

1970   Americans spend $6 billion on **fast food** provided by McDonald's and other fast food chains; by the year 2001, Americans will spend $110 billion a year on fast food, more than on music, videos, newspapers, magazines, movies, and books combined.

1971   An association is found between mothers who took **DES** and a rare form of **vaginal cancer** in their daughters. Apparently the DES taken during pregnancy affected fetal development.

The U.S. Congress declares **war on cancer** with the National Cancer Act; thirty years later, the overall death rate from cancer will remain the same as the date this war was declared.

Japanese food scientists synthesize in a laboratory a **cheaper sweetener called high-fructose corn syrup**, which can be used in frozen foods as protection from freezer burn, as well as in baked goods and vending machine foods to hold freshness. An unanticipated discovery in later years will be that fructose, once consumed, **arrives almost intact in the human liver,** not breaking down. No one can yet guess the health implications.

The United States Department of Agriculture prepares a publication called "An Evaluation of Research in the United States on Human Nutrition; Report No. 2, Benefits from Nutrition Research," which **attributes most major health problems to nutritional deficiencies found in the modern diet.** For twenty-one years this **report will be suppressed from public view**, allegedly at the behest of the food processing industry.

1972   The United States Environmental Protection Agency **bans the pesticide DDT** for its cancer-causing potential in humans.

1973   From this date until 1991, a 126 percent increase in **prostate cancer** will be reported by the National Cancer Institute.

From this date until 1996, **childhood leukemia** will increase 17 percent, **childhood brain cancer** will increase 26 percent,

breast cancer in women will increase 25 percent, and **testicular cancer** will increase 41 percent.

A pediatric allergist tells a conference of the American Medical Association that **food additives** acount for half of the **hyperactivity** cases he sees among his child patients. These children improve dramatically when they no longer consume foods with synthetic colorings, flavors, or preservatives.

The FDA bans the **artificial coloring agent** Violet No. 1 because it is a carcinogen. This **cancer-causing dye** has been used for the previous two decades by the United States Department of Agriculture to stamp every piece of meat sold in the United States with grades of "Prime" or "Choice" or "USDA."

STAGE FOUR: 1974–1997

FOOD QUALITY DETERIORATES

Most meat, fish, and dairy products by the 1970s, if factory farmed, are laced with growth hormones, antibiotics, and a range of pesticides and other toxins. Processed foods have exploded in the sheer numbers of products on grocery store shelves, and most are composed of synthetic chemical additives, such as colorings, preservatives, sugar substitutes, and taste enhancers. Fast food franchises have also emerged as the primary restaurant dining experience for most Americans.

1974   The FDA approves the **artificial sweetener aspartame** after its manufacturer, G.D. Searle & Company, submits study results showing its safety. A year later an FDA task force will find evidence that some of the data submitted by Searle had been **falsified to hide results showing animals fed aspartame had developed seizures and brain tumors,** but no recall or ban will be enacted.

The British physician T.L. Cleave publishes *The Saccharine Disease*, a book that compares disease rates in Western nations with the third world and concludes that **refined carbohydrates** in Western diets contribute to **diabetes and heart disease**.

The FDA **bans the pesticide dieldrin**—in use since the

1920s—as a dangerous carcinogen after lab tests find dieldrin in 96 percent of all meat, fish, and poultry, and 85 percent of all dairy products sold in the nation. Cake mixes and children's cereals are pulled from shelves.

1975   A report by the World Conference on Animal Production estimates that factory-farmed animals contain up to thirty times more **saturated fat** than animals raised just three decades earlier.

1976   The director of the National Cancer Institute, Arthur Upton, tells a committee of the U.S. Congress that half of all **cancers are caused by diet**.

The journal *Scientific American* reports that the diet a **chicken** is placed on in poultry production is "almost totally foreign to any food it ever found in nature. Its feed is a product of the laboratory." This diet includes **antibiotics, hormones**, sulfa drugs, and even arsenic compounds.

1977   The EPA **bans the manufacture and use of PCBs**, citing them as hazardous to human health.

The National Institutes of Health issues the first of **three warnings that an epidemic of obesity is looming** in the United States.

From this date forward to 1994 the number of children in special education programs as a result of **learning disabilities will increase 191 percent**.

1979   **PCBs** are detected in **30 percent of human breast milk**, testing at an average level of 86 parts per billion. This is more than the level of 62.5 ppb that triggers an FDA recall of cow's milk contaminated with PCBs.

1980   From this date until 1992, the **suicide rate** for U.S. teenagers will increase by 30 percent.

From this date to the year 2000, **prescription drug sales will more than triple** to $200 billion a year in the United States, a figure that represents half of all prescription drug sales in the entire world.

Testing by the FDA finds 38 percent of all **grocery foods sampled contain pesticide residues**; by 1998 the FDA will discover that 55 percent of all foods sampled contain pesticides.

1981   As of this date only four out of every ten thousand children in the United States have **autism**, according to the Centers for Disease Control and Prevention. By 1996, the disease will affect thirty-four out of every ten thousand children in the nation.

1982   Teenage boys drink twice as much **milk** as **soda**; within twenty years they will be drinking twice as much soda as milk.

In this year the **bacterium** E. coli 0157:H7 is first identified as **causing illness** and death in humans; it has contaminated live-stock as a result of its concentration in giant feedlots, slaughter-houses, and hamburger grinders.

From this date to 1992, the annual **death rate from asthma** among young people will increase by more than 40 percent.

1983   A neuroscientist writing in *The New England Journal of Medicine* reports that the **artificial sweetener aspartame** may actually in-crease body weight because it stimulates a craving for calorie-laden carbohydrates.

Coke and Pepsi switch from a fifty-fifty mix of sugar and corn syrup in **soft drinks to a 100 percent high-fructose corn syrup sweetener**. Despite evidence that fructose accumulates in the hu-man liver, **no studies have been done** on its long-term safety.

1985   A Smithsonian Institution cancer scientist publishes scientific pa-pers demonstrating that historical outbreaks of **cancer** in fish only began after the widespread distribution of **synthetic chemicals** in the early twentieth century.

The medical journal *The Lancet* reports a study in which 79 percent of **hyperactive** children improve when **artificial color-ings and flavorings** are eliminated from their diet.

Between 1976 and this date, reports the General Accounting Office, **more than half of the 198 drugs approved** by the FDA have turned out to demonstrate **serious health risks**, including organ failure and death.

1986   An estimated 80 percent of **pigs** slaughtered from this date onward will contract **pneumonia** from cramped breeding conditions.

The International Journal of Biosocial Research publishes the re-sults of a four-year study in 803 New York City public schools that found students raised their mean academic scores by 15.7

percent when they were on a diet that **reduced the amounts of artificial food colors, flavors, and preservatives** they consumed in school cafeterias.

1987   A study by the EPA estimates that everyone alive today carries within his or her body at least **seven hundred chemical contaminants**, "most of which have not been well studied."

The National Academy of Sciences releases a report estimating that up to 15 percent of the U.S. population **suffers from multiple chemical sensitivities**, causing various degrees of discomfort; by 1993, just six years later, the academy will estimate that that figure has doubled to 30 percent of the population.

1988   The British medical journal *The Lancet* publishes a study showing a correlation between **vitamin and mineral supplementation and intelligence scores** among British schoolchildren. Dietary deficiencies were found to be hindering school performance.

1989   A division of the National Academy of Sciences warns that the use of antibiotics in factory farms will create **antibiotic-resistant bacteria** that will seriously undermine human health.

A laboratory study in Boston finds that rats given moderate amounts of **fluoride** in their drinking water give birth to **hyperactive babies**, while baby rats exhibit **retardation** and other **cognitive defects**. Many Americans are routinely exposed to higher relative levels of fluoride than the levels administered to the rats.

Tryptophan **supplements genetically engineered** by a Japanese petrochemical company sicken 1,500 people, and forty of them die.

1990   From this date forward, more than one hundred twenty thousand new **processed foods** and beverages will be introduced into a marketplace already filled with three hundred twenty thousand food products competing for shelf space.

As of this date, none of the fifty states has classified 15 percent or more of its population as **obese**; within a decade, all but one state will classify more than 15 percent of its population as obese.

From this date to 1998, the incidence of **diabetes** in the United States will increase by 33 percent.

The FDA discovers that Seldane, an allergy medication, interacts with a variety of other drugs to **create a lethal heart condition**. This discovery is only made as cases of cardiac arrest begin to accumulate.

1991   A vaccinologist warns the president of Merck's vaccine division that six-month-old **children receiving vaccines** containing thimerosal are receiving levels of mercury **eighty-seven times higher** than health guidelines consider safe. Nearly a decade will go by before this pharmaceutical company introduces a mercury-free vaccine to replace thimerosal.

1992   A University of Utah study published in *The Journal of the American Medical Association* finds that water **fluoridation weakens bones** and increases the risk of hip fractures.

The FDA announces a finding that 65 percent of women's **cosmetics** sampled contain **carcinogenic** contaminants.

The Centers for Disease Control and Prevention reports that thirteen thousand patients a year die in the United States from **drug-resistant strains of bacteria**.

Hamburgers at Jack in the Box **fast food** restaurants in the state of Washington are infected with **E. coli** 0157:H7; **four children die** and one hundred more are hospitalized. Only a decade earlier, this strain of E. coli was not even recognized as a hazard to humans. Up to 29 percent of all cattle are thought to be infected by this pathogen as a result of crowded feedlots.

After only four months on the market, the antibiotic Omniflox is withdrawn after **hundreds of adverse reactions are reported**, including multiple organ failures. It is only the ninth drug in FDA history to be withdrawn.

A report in *Annals of Internal Medicine* reveals that 44 percent of **drug ads in medical journals** contain information that would lead physicians to improperly prescribe medications to their patients.

An Earth Summit report issued in Rio de Janeiro warns that farming, grazing, irrigation, and acid rain have **depleted the nutritional minerals in farm and range soils** on every continent of the world over the past one hundred years.

1993   U.S. production of **herbicides** to control unwanted vegetation reaches 750 million pounds a year, or three pounds for every man, woman, and child in the nation.

The FDA approves genetically engineered **bovine growth hormone** (BGH) to increase milk production. Because cows given this hormone develop more frequent udder infections, they are given higher doses of **antibiotics**, which in turn can linger in milk and meat, to be passed on to humans who consume them.

Stanford University School of Medicine researchers report that an **estrogen mimic** called bisphenol A leaks into bottled liquids, such as drinking water, when the **plastic containers** are made of polycarbonates.

Two studies in *The Journal of the American Medical Association* report having examined seventy-four thousand men with vasectomies and finding their **prostate cancer risk** has been increased by up to 66 percent as a result of the procedure.

1994   The U.S. Food and Drug Administration approves the marketing of **genetically modified foods**. Within seven years, genetically modified varieties will account for 26 percent of the corn, 68 percent of the soybeans, and 69 percent of the cotton planted in the United States. Food processors will use ingredients from transgenic corn and soybeans in **60 percent of processed foods** on grocery store shelves.

A **salmonella outbreak** in packaged ice cream sickens more than 220,000 people in forty-one states.

A report by the United States Department of Health and Human Services reveals that the **artificial sweetener aspartame**—a central ingredient in 1,200 food products, including diet drinks—can cause **eighty-eight toxic symptoms** in humans, some of which can lead to death.

The Centers for Disease Control and Prevention report that the **number of low-birth-weight infants rose 6.6 percent** in the United States between 1981 and 1991.

1995   The United States now uses five pounds of **pesticide active ingredients** every year for every person in the nation.

The medical journal *Cancer Causes and Control* reports a USC School of Medicine study in which a higher incidence of leukemia was found in children who ate more than twelve **hot dogs** each month. The trigger for this cancer seemed to be carcinogenic nitrosamines used to preserve **processed meats** used in hot dogs.

1996   An **outbreak of E. coli** O157:H7 in Odwalla **apple juice** hospitalizes seventy people, and one child dies.

Testing of water by the United States Geological Survey finds 95 percent of **water samples** from streams across the United States contain **at least one pesticide**; half of all groundwater wells tested contain pesticide residues.

A **genetically modified tomato** called FlavrSavr is **pulled from the market** only a year after its introduction after studies indicate a problem with low nutritional value and evidence that pathogenic bacteria in human intestines could become antibiotic resistent from the tomato.

1997   A study in the medical journal *Pediatrics* reports the results of a survey of 17,000 girls that finds that **by the age of eight, about one in seven white girls and one out of every two African-American girls are starting puberty**, with breast growth and pubic hair. Even more startling, one out of every one hundred white girls and three out of every one hundred African-American girls show these characteristics at the age of three! The explanation for this **early onset of puberty seems to be in their diets**.

Approved by the FDA just a year earlier, weight-loss drugs Redux and fen-phen are removed from the marketplace after hundreds of reports of **heart valve damage**.

From this date forward, more **prescription drugs** will be declared **toxic** and withdrawn from the marketplace than ever before in history.

A Seattle newspaper breaks the story that **hazardous waste**, including dangerous chemicals and heavy metals, is being recycled into fertilizer and **spread on food crops** across the nation. There is strong evidence the waste enters plant roots and may pose a threat to human health when the plants are eaten.

Testing conducted by the United States Department of Agriculture finds 72 percent of **fruits and vegetables** produced in the

United States contain **detectible levels of pesticides**. One sample of peaches contained the residues of fourteen separate pesticides. A total of ninety-two different pesticides were found in the ten thousand samples of food analyzed by the USDA. DDT was detected in 25 percent of food samples even though it had been banned decades earlier.

STAGE FIVE: 1998–2005

HEALTH IMPACTS ACCELERATE

This period stands out as a watershed stage, revealing the extent of cumulative patterns of health problems associated with synthetic chemicals. Prescription medications are killing more people than ever before. Cases of food-borne diseases are higher than ever before. Vitamin and mineral levels in foods are lower than ever before. More new synthetic chemicals in foods and everyday products are in circulation than ever before.

1998   The FDA withdraws Posicor, a **treatment for angina and hypertension**, after it is revealed to interact dangerously with twenty-five other medications. It has been on the market for less than a year.

The Council for Responsible Nutrition reports that the U.S. health-care system could save $10 billion a year on the costs of treating breast, lung, and stomach **cancers** if only Americans would consume recommended levels of vitamin C, vitamin E, and beta-carotene.

A study published in *The Journal of the American Medical Association* reveals that 106,000 people die each year in American hospitals from the **side effects of prescription medications**. Another 2.2 million people a year have serious but nonfatal reactions to prescribed drugs. Adverse drug reactions have become the fourth leading cause of death in the United States.

As of this date, **75,500 synthetic chemicals** have been registered as appearing in consumer products, agriculture, and industry. The EPA has over 24,000 pesticides registered and the FDA oversees eight thousand chemicals used in cosmetics and as food additives.

The American Journal of Epidemiology publishes a study showing serious negative side effects from chlorine byproducts found in drinking water. Chlorinated tap water in three regions of California **increased miscarriages** among women who drank more **tap water containing chlorine** than bottled water.

1999   According to the Centers for Disease Control and Prevention, the annual reported number of **food-borne disease cases** in the United States amounts to seventy-six million illnesses, three hundred twenty-five thousand hospitalizations, and five thousand deaths. Most are caused by viruses and bacteria.

After forty years of usage, the **antibiotic erythromycin** is linked to serious abdominal obstructions in a study published by the medical journal *The Lancet.*

As of this year, more than **25,000 cosmetics chemicals** are in use. Less than 4 percent of these cosmetics ingredients have been tested for safety in humans.

The United States Public Health Service issues a warning that **routine vaccinations are exposing many infants to quantities of mercury** well above safe levels. The mercury is in the form of thimerosal, an antibacterial additive in many childhood vaccines.

2000   The National Academy of Sciences reports that **half of all pregnancies** in the United States result in less-than-healthy babies. Up to one-third of the developmental defects in these babies are caused by exposure to toxic chemicals.

Half of all Americans now take at least one prescription drug every day; 25 percent of Americans take **multiple prescription drugs** every day.

The incidence of **testicular cancer** is now estimated to be **four times higher** than just fifty years earlier.

The medical journal *Primary Psychiatry* reports that after five decades of usage, the drug Mellaril has been linked to **heart damage**. This problem with the drug was first identified thirty years earlier.

The American Journal of Epidemiology reports that after five decades of usage, the **antidepressants** imipramine and amitriptyline are associated with increased rates of **breast cancer**.

Three drugs previously approved by the FDA—Lotronex for irritable bowel, Propulsid for heartburn, and Rezulin for diabetes— are **withdrawn** after patients experience intestinal damage, heart arrhythmia, and liver toxicity.

Physicians for Social Responsibility releases a report describing "an **epidemic of developmental, learning and behavioral disabilities**" affecting an estimated twelve million children in the United States. Evidence suggests the epidemic may be a result of **toxic chemicals** affecting the central nervous systems of these children.

University of Toronto researchers feed hamsters a **high-fructose diet** (similar to soft drinks and processed foods containing corn syrup) to mimic the diet of young adult humans. The hamsters have a metabolism similar to humans. Within a few weeks the hamsters develop **high triglyceride levels in the blood, and insulin resistance**.

2001   The Centers for Disease Control and Prevention announces that the **food** we eat is responsible for twice the numbers of **illnesses** in the United States in comparison to just seven years earlier.

The New England Journal of Medicine reports that **80 percent of meat** packages containing beef, chicken, or pork sampled from supermarkets are **infected with bacteria resistant to antibiotics** and, once consumed, will survive in human intestines for up to a week.

About **25 percent of children under age nineteen in the United States are overweight**; this figure has doubled in the past 30 years.

The Journal of the American Medical Association publishes a study revealing that of 6.7 million adult annual visits to the doctor for a sore throat between 1989 and 1999, **antibiotics were prescribed in 73 percent of the visits even though antibiotics do not treat viral infections**.

2002   *The Journal of the American Medical Association* reports a relationship between **chronic disease** and vitamin intake, recommending that all adults take at least one multivitamin a day because the absence of these **vitamins** in their food puts them at risk for cancer, cardiovascular disease, and osteoporosis.

The U.S. **pharmaceutical industry now employs** 675 lobbyists, including 26 former members of Congress, and spends $91 million a year on influencing decisions made by Congress.

The combined **profits** of the **ten largest U.S. drug companies** reach $35.9 billion, a sum higher than the combined profits for all the other 490 corporations on the Fortune 500 list of largest corporations.

Of the seventy-eight "new" drugs approved by the FDA in this year, only seventeen contain new active molecular ingredients, and **only 7** of these, according to the FDA, are actually **improvements over older drugs** already on the market.

For the first time since 1958, the U.S. **infant mortality rate increases**. It is now twice that of Japan and most other industrial nations.

McDonald's now operates thirty thousand fast food restaurants in one hundred countries. Each day, **one in four Americans visits a fast food restaurant**.

The Centers for Disease Control and Prevention reports a study in which 289 persons were tested and **in every one of their bodies** was found the plasticizer dibutyl phthalate (DBP), a toxic **ingredient used in cosmetics**, primarily nail polish.

2003   As of this date, 80 percent of the soy and 38 percent of the corn planted in the United States are **genetically engineered**; derivatives of these two crops now show up in 70 percent of all **processed foods**.

The Centers for Disease Control and Prevention reports that of all babies born in the United States in 2000, at least **one-third will become diabetics**.

Harvard School of Public Health researchers report in the journal *Epidemiology* that phthalates found in plastics may be contributing to **reproductive defects**. The study of 168 male patients at a fertility clinic found that the men with the highest levels of phthalates in their blood were also those with the lowest sperm counts and lowest sperm vitality.

2004   The **arthritis drug** Vioxx is ordered off the market by the FDA after thousands of people experience **strokes and heart attacks**. The British medical journal *The Lancet* declares that the FDA should have withdrawn the drug four years earlier based on the negative results of twenty-nine clinical trials.

The science journal *Public Health* prints a study revealing that the incidence of **death from brain diseases**, such as Alzheimer's and Parkinson's, **more than tripled** during the period of 1974 to 1997.

The science journal *Environmental Science & Technology* reveals that a **toxic chemical flame retardant**, PBDE, used in carpeting, electronics, and furniture, has **contaminated thirty-one of thirty-two common name-brand groceries** tested, including ice cream, eggs, milk, butter, cheese, chicken, and turkey.

Research published in *The Journal of the American Medical Association* reveals that within a year of arriving in the United States, 16 percent of **new immigrants become obese** for the first time in their lives.

The **pesticide diazinon**, sold in the United States for a half-century as a lawn, garden, and household bug-killer, is **banned** by the EPA after it is found to be a toxic threat to children who encounter it, damaging their nervous systems.

A study in *The Journal of the American Heart Association* reveals that over the previous decade the number of adults with **high blood pressure increased by 30 percent**.

A study in the medical journal *Archives of Disease in Childhood* reveals that four hundred children were tested for the effects of **food additives and artificial preservatives** on their behavior. The results demonstrated "a substantial effect" of these synthetics **stimulating hyperactivity and behavioral problems**.

Stanford University biologists report that **musk fragrances**, used to improve the smell of **detergents, soaps, air fresheners, shampoos, perfumes, and colognes**, escape unscathed from municipal sewage treatment processes and **accumulate in the tissues of fish, mussels, and other invertebrates.** Japan previously banned musk xylene as a toxic threat to humans.

2005   The FDA rules that **advertising** for the arthritis drugs Bextra and Celebrex must be withdrawn for being **misleading and unsubstantiated,** after a study finds Celebrex, made by Pfizer, increases the risk of **heart attacks.**

The FDA announces that it is issuing **twice the number of public advisories about drug risks and adding five times as many black box warnings** on drug labels as it did just a year earlier.

Two science studies in the journal *Circulation* turn up evidence that the **entire class of painkillers known as COX-2 inhibitors puts users at risk of heart attacks and strokes.** The drugs studied were Bextra and Celebrex, both of which remain on the market.

United States Geological Survey scientists in Colorado discover that the by-products of antibacterial soap, prescription drugs, steroids, bug spray, and other **chemical products** are entering streams and groundwater and **disrupting fish reproduction while increasing resistance to antibiotics** among people who consume the fish.

An American Heart Association journal reveals that middle-aged men with high levels of mercury in their bodies have a **70 percent increased risk of death by heart disease.** The primary source of their **mercury contamination** is fish that absorbed the toxins from power plants, factories, and other industrial operations that use chlorine. **Fetuses and children are also particularly vulnerable.**

The medical journal *Cancer Epidemiology Biomarkers and Prevention* reports a Columbia University study examining the health effects of exposure of pregnant women to **air pollutants** in New York City. A **50 percent increase in the level of persistent genetic abnormalities in infants** was detected in those whose mothers had high air pollution exposure.

Breast milk sampled from women in **eighteen states** is found to **contain traces of perchlorate, a toxic component of rocket**

fuel. Texas Tech University researchers report the source is likely to be food that was tainted from irrigation water that had collected the toxin in seepage from defense industry plants around the United States. At levels found in the breast milk, a one-month-old infant would absorb enough perchlorate to exceed safe levels set by a panel of the National Academy of Sciences.

The journal *Health Affairs* reports that about **half of all personal bankruptcies that occur each year in the United States are due to medical bills**. An estimated two million people experience personal bankruptcy due to catastropic illness.

Yale School of Medicine researchers report that low doses of the environmental contaminant bisphenol A (BPA), used to make many plastics found in **food storage containers**, can **lead to learning disabilities in children and neurodegenerative diseases in adults**.

An independent scientific advisory board to the EPA issues a draft report finding that a **toxic chemical found on the coatings of take-out food containers**—perfluorooctanoic sulfuric acid—is being found widely in human blood tests across the United States. This chemical is likely to **cause cancer in humans**.

Researchers at Virginia Tech University find evidence that a variety of consumer products, such as some toothpastes, dishwashing liquids, and antimicrobial soaps, produce **chloroform gas** when the triclosan in these products reacts with chlorinated water. Chloroform **can cause depression, liver problems, and cancer when inhaled or absorbed through the skin**.

The FDA reports that two thousand women who used the **acne drug Accutane** while pregnant either had **miscarriages or abortions** because the drug caused severe birth defects in the fetuses.

Surgical clinics surveyed by *The Sunday Times* in Britain report **a sharp upsurge in the number of men seeking breast reduction surgery**. Hormones in the water are blamed for a doubling of cases in just a year of gynecomastia, a hormone-induced growth of men's breasts.

The FDA posts a warning that the popular antidepressant Paxil may **increase the risk of birth defects** if pregnant women take it during the first trimester of pregnancy.

An independent advisory committee to the FDA warns that **antibacterial soaps are no more effective** than common soap in reducing illness from bacteria and are dangerous because the antibacterial chemicals contribute to bacterial resistance to antibiotics.

The FDA warns doctors that children and adolescents who take the drug Strattera to treat attention deficit/hyperactivity disorder may experience **increased suicidal thoughts and may attempt suicide as a result**.

Researchers with the Southern California Coastal Water Research Project discover that two-thirds of some species of fish examined from coastal waters off Los Angeles and Orange counties possess **both male and female reproductive organs**. The seafloor sediment in these areas is **contaminated with estrogenic chemicals** from wastewater effluent generated by nine million inhabitants of coastal cities.

Researchers at the University of Copenhagen report in *Environmental Health Perspectives* that **human development is vulnerable to the phthalates** found in plastics from everyday products. Of ninety-six baby boys studied, those with the least testosterone had the highest levels of exposure to phthalates found in their mothers' breast milk.

A report by the Government Accountability Office, the investigative arm of Congress, finds that the EPA is **failing to protect people from tens of thousands of toxic chemicals**. Chemical companies have provided health impact data to the EPA for only about 15 percent of chemicals introduced over the past thirty years.

In the largest study of chemical exposure ever conducted on humans, the Centers for Disease Control and Prevention finds more than **one hundred toxic substances in the bodies of the 2,400 people tested**. Children are found to carry higher levels of these synthetic chemicals in their bodies than adults.

The United States spends more than **twice as much on health care** than any other industrialized nation in the world—$6,100 per year for every man, woman, and child. Fifteen percent of the economy is now devoted to medical care, up from 10 percent in 1987. Yet, the United States ranks forty-sixth in life expectancy and forty-second in infant mortality among the nations of the world.

One of the more obvious recurring patterns that emerges from reading the Slippery Slope Index is how often harm is inflicted on human health because of insufficient testing of new chemicals, especially testing of the long-term health effects. As we will see in Part II, entrenched institutional forces within the economy and government cooperate to keep the public largely unaware of the extent to which a toxic threat exists within their foods and medicines.

PART TWO

STRANGERS IN A STRANGE LAND

Our Rapid Decline

Pharmaceutical drugs are prescribed to mask our symptoms in the hope that, with time, our immune systems will do the actual healing.

But our immune systems are being compromised by inadequate nutrition, overuse of antibiotics, and the chemical toxins our bodies absorb and store.

We pass these immune system—weakening traits on to our offspring while they are still in the womb.

While we pretend that everything is normal, our toxic chemical legacy is producing ever-greater numbers of genetic defects in our species and in the animal life that surrounds us.

CHAPTER FOUR

WIZARDS OF OZ: THE FOOD INDUSTRY

". . . the choices you make each day in something as fundamental as what you eat have consequences that are far-reaching, not only for yourself but also for a much wider society."

—Dean Ornish in his foreword to *The Food Revolution*, by John Robbins

LET'S THROW A DINNER PARTY

You decide to host a dinner party and invite a half dozen of your friends, neighbors, or relatives to a meal you will prepare in your kitchen. Let's say it's a mainstream American meal of roast beef, pan-fried potatoes, and sweet bell peppers stuffed with cheese, accompanied by a spinach salad, bread with butter or margarine, and peach cobbler for dessert. You give your guests a drink choice of either iced tea or soda.

At the surface level the meal you prepare will look and smell and taste wonderfully appetizing and nutritious. But let's say you are also a stranger in a strange land and you are curious to probe beneath these surface appearances, all the way down to the molecular level. You don't want to be neurotic about it; you just want to be informed. So you begin to ask some questions, do some research, and here is what you find.

Let's start with the potatoes. As you fry them in a Teflon skillet you release molecules of the indestructible Teflon chemicals into your food and into the air. The potatoes themselves are already contaminated with a half dozen pesticide residues that your vigorous washing fails to remove because the pesticides penetrated into the potatoes' skin. So now you have heated the Teflon and pesticide molecules into a frenzied mixture that no one may have ever studied for impacts on human health.

You make the tea using tap water containing chlorine, fluoride, and molecules of perchlorate, a chemical used in rocket fuel, flares, and air bags that now commonly shows up in tap water. This water also contains by-products of chlorination, including trihalomethanes and haloacetic acids, which have been linked to cancer, reproductive problems, and birth defects. Your guests add an artificial sweetener containing the synthetic chemical aspartame to their tea. This chemical also appears in all of the sodas. (Much more about aspartame later in this chapter.)

Both the spinach and the lettuce you use for the salad contain traces of perchlorate, that pesky rocket fuel that migrates everywhere. The spinach also hides traces of up to ten separate pesticides, if we are to believe food-testing surveys. Those bell peppers you serve contain residues of up to nine pesticides. The salad dressing everyone uses contains a collection of chemicals that act as preservatives, colorings, flavorings, and artificial sweeteners.

Your beef, which everyone feasts on, was raised in a gigantic factory farm feedlot where thousands of cows are crowded together and fed growth hormones, appetite stimulants, antibiotics, and tranquilizers, chemicals that become a body burden in the animals' flesh. Their feed was intentionally laced with other synthetic chemicals and unintentionally contaminated with residues of insecticides and herbicides. These animals have passed traces of their body burden on to you.

The bread you serve contains flour that the manufacturer has aged using oxidizing agents such as chlorine. The chlorine was blasted onto the flour during the final stage of production, and some chlorine molecules survived the bread's baking process. Many European countries, Germany being one, banned the use of chlorine as an oxidizing agent for bread a half century ago, fearing the impacts on health.

The margarine your guests spread on this bread contains trans fats that raise cholesterol and contribute to heart disease. A by-product of the hy-drogenation process for margarine is a residue of toxic metals, such as nickel and aluminum, left behind in the finished product. You can visual-ize margarine's effect on your body simply by leaving a cube of it sitting out on a counter for several months—it will not be touched by mold, in-sects, or rodents. If you use butter on your bread instead of margarine, you eat one of the most contaminated food items of all, because cows of-fload some of their own body burdens of toxins into their milk.

You pull the peach cobbler out of the refrigerator and stick it into the microwave to heat it in preparation for serving. The cobbler is inside a plastic container, and the act of microwaving that container releases the chemical DEHA into the cobbler. DEHA is a plasticizer that the EPA la-bels a possible human carcinogen. But there is another unexpected prob-lem with the cobbler. You use peaches contaminated with up to nine separate pesticide residues, which have penetrated the skin. No one knows if synergies are created when the high heat of microwaves combines pesti-cide residues with migrating molecules of plastics. If you decide to add a scoop of vanilla ice cream to the cobbler, you probably will ingest dioxin, a toxic bioaccumulative chemical that is sometimes found in ice cream at levels up to two hundred times greater than what the EPA considers safe.

If you had served veal rather than plain old beef during this meal, the calves would have been raised on diets designed to keep them anemic but still alive and treated with antibiotics and other drugs, two being nitro-furazone (a known carcinogen), and chloramphenicol (which can cause blood disorders in some humans). No one knows the long-term health consequences or the synergistic effects in the human body of consuming cow flesh containing such a heavy body burden of chemicals.

Eating chicken would have done little to lessen the hazards. A *Scien-tific American* article back in 1976 raised the first alert about poultry pro-duction chemical practices when it revealed how the chicken we consume is raised "on a diet almost totally foreign to any food it ever found in na-ture. Its feed is a product of the laboratory." These laboratory creations for the chicken diet include antibiotics, sulfa drugs, hormones, and even ar-senic compounds.

Had you selected fish for the meal you would have needed to avoid shark, swordfish, king mackerel, and tilefish because these types of fish have been found to carry the heaviest loads of toxic metals. So what about pork? Consumer champion John Robbins noted in his book *Diet For a New America* how pork production relies upon a range of synthetic chemicals, such as a feed additive for fertility, XLP-30, produced by Shell Oil. It is given to sows to increase their birth rate. A Shell official conceded the depth of our collective ignorance about the health implications by saying, "we don't know why it works."

Throughout the twentieth century severe outbreaks of diseases and illnesses emerged at the same time that we began to experience sharp declines in the nutritional quality of our foods. Also, it was no coincidence that this period happened to be when we were first subjected to an avalanche of chemical additives in a wide array of processed food products. This pattern of interconnections is one of the key distinguishing features of the Hundred-Year Lie. Let's dissect it, beginning with the health symptoms.

WE HAVE BECOME WHAT WE EAT

When nineteen-year-old Florida college student Jordan Rubin came down with his sickness, symptoms manifested suddenly on a summer afternoon in 1994. He felt fatigue accompanied by stomach cramps, nausea, and diarrhea. In just a week he shed twenty pounds. Every night he battled 104-degree fevers that, when combined with hourly trips to the bathroom, induced severe sleep deprivation. Within months he was so emaciated, he resembled a concentration camp prisoner. He was diagnosed with Crohn's disease, an "incurable" degenerative disease of the intestinal tract.

Over the next two years his health continued to deteriorate until he was in a wheelchair. He consulted seventy health practitioners from seven countries and tried every imaginable form of therapy, all without finding permanent relief or a cure. Along the way, he made some alarming discoveries about the standards of Western medicine and about the levels of nutrition in our nation's food supply.

"So much of what passes for scientifically validated nutritional supplementation . . . has little, if any, scientific substance," Jordan concluded. "I was going to have to take medication if I wanted to stay alive. Yet, the side effects of the medications that keep you alive can be almost as bad as the disease itself."

Finally in 1996, Jordan found a nutritionist with a program that sounded rather strange, to say the least, but which Jordan intuitively felt was worth trying. The nutritionist counseled Jordan to adopt the diet of his ancestors, the ancient Israelites. This diet had an emphasis on consuming living foods that were rich with beneficial microorganisms. He was told that these living microorganisms and trace minerals are nutrients that have been mostly eliminated from our modern, pesticide-sterilized soils and pasteurized food products.

Using a bag of these soil organisms, Jordan created additives for a daily diet that also included yeast-free whole grains, organic fruits, vegetables, and other " 'live' foods with their beneficial enzymes and microorganisms intact." Within a month this black powder of soil organisms had given Jordan new bursts of energy, and he gained twenty-nine pounds. By the end of 1996, he had returned to his normal weight before the illness. He felt healthy again. Jordan deduced that health can be improved through whole-food nutrition and whole-food supplements, which bring us back to a diet and a lifestyle that have been proven to work for thousands of years. He eventually became a consumer activist and wrote several books conveying a health message based on his experience.

Probiotics is now a widely accepted medical term referring to the beneficial bacteria that support digestion and help to keep us healthy. Both poor diets and chemical toxins, especially pharmaceutical drugs, deplete levels of these good bacteria in the body.

Jordan's health crisis may seem unusual and abnormally severe, yet it illustrates the range of health effects traceable to a food supply that has been depleted of its nutrients, loaded with synthetic chemicals, and stripped of its health-protective value. The health benefits of literally eating dirt for the content of essential minerals may be making a comeback in some surprising ways.

A compulsion to consume clay or dirt has traditionally been viewed by Western medicine as a symptom of mental illness if it occurs in adults rather than children. It even has a clinical name as a malady—geophagy.

Now some medical experts are acknowledging there may be health benefits to eating clay or dirt, especially for pregnant women, because the compulsion is a natural body response to deficiencies in the mineral content of our food and the body's need to expel chemical toxins.

"Soil is nature's multimineral supply," says David L. Katz, a nutrition expert at the Yale School of Medicine, "and nature favors behaviors that lead to survival. . . . It is possible that the binding effect of clay would cause it to absorb toxins."

These physical cravings some people experience for calcium, iron, copper, and magnesium—some of the very essential minerals for the immune system—are a result of these minerals having been leached from the food crops sold in supermarkets. Magnesium is important to the functioning of at least three hundred enzymes in the body, many of which are crucial to the body's ability to detoxify synthetic chemicals.

To understand how drastically the nutrient levels in our food have fallen, we need only examine the Department of Agriculture's own statistical measurements. USDA nutrition information reveals that between 1973 and 1997, for every vegetable grown in the United States, every single nutrient that can be measured in each category of vegetable has undergone huge declines. For raw broccoli, average calcium levels dropped 53 percent in that time frame, riboflavin declined 48 percent, thiamine nosedived 35 percent, and niacin 29 percent. Similar nutrient declines were found for cabbage, carrots, cauliflower, onions, and a long list of others.

While admitting their own data revealed the declines, USDA officials nonetheless tried to explain away these embarrassing losses of nutrient values in food by claiming that "testing techniques have simply become more accurate, making the old data wrong." This was the sort of rationalization that I heard repeatedly in researching this book, whether it was from,the chemical industry claiming that statistical evidence revealing a higher incidence of various diseases was due to "more sensitive and accurate tests to detect the diseases," or the medical and pharmaceutical industries dismissing the health impact of chemical synergies because "our most sophisticated testing can't detect them," as if somehow it made sense that something we can't measure must not exist.

To dissect the USDA contention that more accurate testing accounts for the decline in food nutrients, a group of scientists took the measuring technology that the USDA used back in 1973 and applied it to some contemporary crops of vegetables. They found that the 1973 measurement technology detected only 6 percent less calcium or other nutrients than did the 1997 technology used by the USDA, making it clear that technology alone couldn't begin to account for the tremendous declines in the nutrient values of our food.

HOW WE LOST THE NUTRIENTS

Most large grocery chains these days post a sign in at least one section of their stores describing it as a "health food" section, which has prompted some of us to wonder whether the rest of the supermarket should have signs identifying aisles as filled with "illness food," or "unhealthy food," or even "death food."

The somewhat arbitrary distinctions being drawn by the food industry between what is supposedly healthy and unhealthy prompted me to ask which basic nutrients our bodies really need from food to maintain a naturally occurring state of health. There is an emerging consensus about the answer, and it relies upon an understanding of our genetic history and nature.

What we humans consume for food has undergone more profound change in the past century than in the previous one hundred thousand years, yet genetically we have the same bodies and nutritional needs as our hunter-gatherer ancestors. That discrepancy between who we are and what we put into our bodies has sown the seeds for our current epidemics of illness and disease.

The argument that our modern, processed-foods diet, laced with synthetic chemicals, is at odds with the diet we're genetically programmed to follow was advanced in 1985 by S. Boyd Eaton in a scientific paper he published in *The New England Journal of Medicine*. The idea was more fully developed by Loren Cordain, professor in the health and exercise science department at Colorado State University, writing in his 2002 book, *The Paleo Diet*. "Our genes determine our nutritional needs," wrote

Cordain, and "many modern foods are at odds with our genetic makeup," a situation that is "the cause of many of our modern diseases."

Long before Cordain and Eaton introduced their food and health ideas, an American dentist named Weston A. Price spent the 1930s traveling with his wife among isolated tribes and peoples throughout the world—from Peru to the Congo to Fiji—studying the relationships between their diet, nutrition, and overall health. He found fourteen tribal diets that afforded virtual immunity to tooth decay, illness, and disease. What these diverse diets had in common was that not a single one contained any processed foods or hydrogenated vegetable oils, and each diet had four times the quantity of minerals and water-soluble vitamins that could be found in the diets of any industrialized country at that time.

In his 1939 book, *Nutrition and Physical Degeneration,* Price described how nutritional diets common among tribal peoples endowed them with strong teeth and strong physiques, but both conditions quickly deteriorated once they were exposed to processed foods. He found a direct correlation between the mineral depletion of soils and nutritional imbalances in people. He also may have been the first to write about the importance of food synergies to health.

"We have used our scientific knowledge largely to change nature's foods and thereby have defeated nature's laws of health," said Price. "Nature has put foods up in packages containing the combinations of minerals and other factors that are essential for nourishing the various organs. Our modern process of robbing the natural foods for convenience or gain completely thwarts nature's inviolable program."

Our food-crop soils have become anemic, stripped of the ninety or so nutrients essential to human health as a result of fertilizers, pesticides, herbicides, irrigation, acid rain, and other related factors. Nutrient deficiencies that result in the human body depress and kill cells in the immune system, rendering the body more vulnerable to illness and disease. "There is increasing evidence that our more polluted environment in combination with a poorer, nutrient-deficient diet is damaging our immune systems," reports Paula Baillie-Hamilton.

An Earth Summit report issued in 1992 estimated that 85 percent of nutrients were removed from crop soils in North America during the twentieth century. Other parts of the world fared little better—Asia and

South America both lost 76 percent of nutrients from soils, Africa lost 74 percent, and Europe declined 72 percent.

Nutrition expert Joel D. Wallach breaks the ninety-one nutrients essential to human health down this way—sixty minerals, sixteen vitamins, twelve amino acids, and three essential fatty acids, which together are required daily for optimal health and longevity. "The entire complement of the ninety-one essential nutrients required historically found in our earthly foods are no longer there—they are either totally absent or their availability is so highly variable that your chances of obtaining them from food alone is more of a gamble than a Las Vegas crapshoot!"

Processing food removes even more nutrients. Consider what happens with canned tuna. The canning process removes 99 percent of vitamin A found in fresh tuna, 97 percent of vitamin B_1, 86 percent of vitamin B_2, and 45 percent of niacin, and it increases the level of oxidized cholesterol in the human body. Oxidized cholesterol is a substance "routinely fed to laboratory animals to accelerate artery clogging in order to test theories of heart disease," reports nutrition expert Loren Cordain. When whole wheat is refined into white flour for white bread, the percentage and range of nutrients lost are extraordinary: fiber, 95 percent; iron, 84 percent; vitamin E, 95 percent; manganese, 82 percent; niacin, 80 percent; vitamin B_2, 81 percent. Many foods and spices are also irradiated to neutralize insects and microorganisms, but this process further destroys vitamins and other essential nutrients in the food and eliminates the soil organisms that produce natural antibiotic compounds.

In an attempt to compensate for nutrient losses at every step of the food-production and -manufacturing process, food processors have resorted to synthetic food additives, the so-called functional foods. "Fortification permits manufacturers to market foods of dubious nutritional quality as health foods—even to health professionals," writes Marion Nestle, a professor of nutrition at New York University and author of *Food Politics*. She cites an advertisement that appeared in the *American Journal of Public Health* in 1999 from the Kellogg's cereal company: "Froot Loops cereal? . . . presweetened cereals are a major source of nutrients for kids in the U.S."

"No functional food can ever replace the full range of nutrients and phytochemicals present in fruits, vegetables, and whole grains," counters

Nestle, "nor can they overcome the detrimental effects of diets that are not already healthful."

As far back as 1926, a United States Department of Commerce consumer survey showed that most Americans preferred fresh products over processed foods, based on flavor and nutritional value. But 100 percent of those surveyed also agreed that canned foods were more convenient, and as a result they were willing to sacrifice taste and nutrition to lessen preparation time.

"American food processing became more complex and the wizardry of food chemists rivaled the ancient dreams of alchemists, turning the pedestrian contents of their beakers into substances that looked and tasted like sugar, bacon, cream, and other delights," wrote Harvey Levenstein in his wonderful history of food, *Revolution at the Table.* "There was little inclination to question the products of the food business, which seemed to be making life easier for the housewife with each new chemical breakthrough."

What most profoundly changed the eating habits of Americans and then the world was that chemical concoction known as the TV dinner. Though the United States Army and an airline food service company actually invented the concept, it was the CA Swanson & Sons company that popularized it in the early 1950s, with trays of frozen turkey, sweet potatoes, and peas inadvertently creating the fast food industry and with it, the necessity for someone to invent the microwave oven.

These advances were heralded as extraordinary triumphs of the atomic age. Now, fast-forward to what we confront today. As I write these words I have just read an article about another new chemical that tricks the taste buds into sensing salt or sugar without those substances actually being there. Invented by a biotechnology company in conjunction with Kraft, Nestle, Coca-Cola, and the Campbell Soup company, this new chemical has no flavor of its own and because it falls under the category of artificial flavor, it can be placed into food products without being listed on the ingredient label. The four food companies have contracted exclusive rights to use this new chemical but, citing trade secrecy laws, they refuse to identify what products will contain it. They insist that even without testing it they know this chemical will be safe for human consumption because it will be used in tiny quantities.

Nothing in the realm of food turns out to be quite as it seems. Take the Natural Flavors Illusion. There is no real difference between "natural flavor" and "artificial flavor" on any list of food ingredients. Both categories represent synthetic chemicals produced by slightly different methods. Most every product labeled sugar free, diet, or low calorie contains chemical additives and artificial sweeteners that lull us into thinking they are somehow more healthy than what they replaced. This has become a recurring pattern in the food land of Oz. For example, we were told for decades by "food authorities" and food processors that lab-created margarine was healthier for us than natural butter. Then decades later it was discovered that the hydrogenated oils in margarine contribute to heart disease, and so margarine was less healthy than butter after all.

MYTHS WE CHERISH

FOOD ADDITIVES ARE HARMLESS

Humans have used naturally occurring additives throughout recorded history to preserve food and enhance its taste. Salt was used by our ancestors to preserve fish and meats, sugar helped to preserve fruit, and vinegar was used to pickle vegetables. Spices and herbs were added to improve the flavors of foods, and that became the foundation of our many culinary traditions.

Today's food additives are almost completely products of chemical laboratories and are extraordinarily effective at what they do. Adding synthetic chemicals directly to our food was done to satisfy a mixture of public needs and industry intentions. These chemicals preserve foodstuffs for extended periods, which prolongs shelf life to the public's benefit. They enhance the taste and texture of food as compensation for what is lost in processing. And finally, as a Trojan horse financial benefit to food manufacturers, the additives stimulate your appetite (and body chemistry) so you will consume more of the product.

Additives are ingeniously designed. Food product texture and consistency are maintained by adding chemical ingredients as emulsifiers, stabilizers, and thickeners. Preservatives have been created, such as BHA and

BHT, that dramatically slow spoilage and rancidity. Chemical additives give the food pleasing colors, appearances, aromas, and added flavors. Other chemicals are leavening agents or help to control acidity and alkalinity in foods. It is all really quite impressive, and the chemical creations only seem limited by the human imagination.

Ingredient companies sell $4 billion worth of these additives to the food processing industry each year, and these chemicals, or variations of them, show up in practically every processed food product, as well as in many fast foods. The artificial tastes and aromas in processed and fast foods are mostly a product of a few large chemical plant laboratories off the New Jersey turnpike. In his book *Fast Food Nation*, Eric Schlosser demonstrated how the flavor and aroma industries grew out of the already established perfume industry.

"In addition to being the world's largest flavor company," wrote Schlosser, "IFF manufactures the smell of six of the ten best-selling fine perfumes in the United States. . . . It also makes the smell of household products such as deodorant, dishwashing detergent, bath soap, shampoo, furniture polish, and floor wax. All of these aromas are made through the same basic process: the manipulation of volatile chemicals to create a particular smell. The basic science behind the scent of your shaving cream is the same as that governing the flavor of your TV dinner."

Everyone naturally wants to believe additives are safe and that industry scientists and government regulators are vigorously testing each and every potential threat before that threat hurts someone. But what evidence do we have for feeling reassured?

A revealing insight comes from a brochure published in 2000 by a food industry group, the International Food Information Council. In the midst of rhetorical arguments that artificial additives are as safe as natural additives, out pops this admission: "Of the original two hundred provisionally listed color additives, ninety have been listed as safe and the remainder have either been removed from use by FDA or withdrawn by industry."

Let's digest the preceding. We have just learned that more than half of all synthetic colorings are dangerous to health and have been taken off the market. These colorings are usually made from coal tar dyes commonly found in fabrics, paints, and inks, and yet they have been added to processed foods and been consumed for years by millions of people. When were the additives taken out of circulation? After the humans who had been consuming them became sick or died, or after some conscience-ridden scientist decided to test on lab animals what humans were being subjected to. It seems that safety concerns about food additives are mostly an afterthought dependent on how the human guinea pigs react.

Ross Hume Hall, professor emeritus of biochemistry at Canada's Mc-Master University, put it this way: "The safety of a food additive is not something you can personally check. It takes sophisticated laboratories and technical knowledge to do the testing. So you depend on the government to ensure that the testing is done. Yet the federal government allows thousands of chemical additives in your food that have not been tested for safety. When you take a bite of commercial food containing food additives, foreign chemicals enter your body whose safety was approved with 1930s knowledge."

Consider another category of food additives, artificial flavors, which are usually added to replace more expensive ingredients in some products or to obscure the bland or poor taste of highly processed foods. Of the more than two thousand chemicals used in various combinations to produce specific flavors, few have been researched or tested to determine individual effects on health, much less the possible synergistic effects inside the human body. At least one hundred new synthetic additives are added to the food supply each year.

Can chemical food ingredients alter brain chemistry? Are toxic thoughts and actions the result of toxic meals? Can irritability, aggressiveness, impulsiveness, and other behaviors be traced to the accumulation of food toxins in our bodies, especially children's bodies?

Only within the last two decades of the twentieth century did such questions assume relevance to a generation of parents and teachers who began witnessing an unprecedented wave of attention, learning, and behavioral disorders among children. Look at what is happening around us, to our children, to ourselves.

"School children struggle with their homework because they can't remember or focus," writes clinical nutritionist Carol Simontacchi in her

2001 book, *The Crazy Makers*. "They fight anger that bubbles up from nowhere and scalds the people they love most dearly. They find themselves fighting irrational fears that hinder them in relationships, schools, and on the job. We've been told over and over that our food choices are contributing to degenerative diseases like cancer, diabetes, and heart disease. Maybe it's time that we explore the possiblity that these major American consumer brand 'foods' are destroying our brains, too. Cell by cell."

The number of kids in the United States and Britain being administered Ritalin and other drugs for hyperactivity and related disorders has more than tripled in the past few decades. By even the most conservative estimates, up to 6 percent of U.S. schoolchildren suffer the health disorder called ADD—attention deficit disorder. Another 20 percent of students seem to exhibit some form of behavioral problems. Suicide rates are way up, and even the childhood homicide rate in the United States is five times the rate of any other industrialized country.

It was as if this epidemic of scrambled brain chemistry came out of nowhere. But if you were to chart on a graph the incidence of these disorders, you would find a corresponding increase in the numbers and levels of chemical additives in the foods and drinks these children consumed.

If our bodies are like giant chemistry sets, then our brains are chemical factories, sensitive to every foreign chemical hitchhiking through our blood. "Some of these chemicals are quite toxic to the brain," says Russell Blaylock, a neurosurgeon and expert on the human brain and nervous system. "For example, glutamate can cause widespread destruction of certain brain cells in concentrations normally found in the diet. This is especially so when we consider the enormous amounts of glutamate added to our food in the form of the taste enhancer MSG."

Animal studies have shown that MSG can stimulate the release of hormones throughout the body, and lab animals exposed to MSG become grossly obese and experience difficulty in sexual reproduction. By some estimates the amount of MSG added to the typical restaurant meal, especially Chinese cuisine, can amount to nine grams for a single dish, enough to cause brain damage in lab animals. It is commonly added to most Kentucky Fried Chicken, McDonald's, Taco Bell, and other fast food products, as well as to most frozen foods.

In fact, when scientists need to create obese rats or mice for their diabetes test studies, they inject the animals with MSG soon after birth. This MSG triples the amount of insulin produced by the pancreas, and the rodents rapidly grow fat. If you do an Internet search of the National Library of Medicine database, looking under MSG and obesity, you will find many dozens of science studies drawing a link between MSG use and weight gain. There is a growing body of evidence that MSG is one of the synthetic chemical substances that can trigger diabetes in humans.

Excitotoxins is the term Blaylock used as the title of a 1997 book exposing the dangers of MSG, aspartame, and a whole class of other food additives whose only purpose is to enhance the taste of foods that lack nutrition, such as potato chips, soft drinks, frozen foods, and diet foods. Both MSG and aspartame now appear in so many processed food products that a complete list would either bore or frighten you to death. Quite often food labels will say "no MSG" or "no MSG added" when in fact MSG is present, piggybacking as part of other ingredients in the list. Sometimes MSG is hidden on the label under the term hydrolyzed vegetable protein or under natural meat tenderizer.

Research referenced by Blaylock indicates that both glutamate and aspartame not only can excite neurons in the brain until these cells degenerate and die, but these chemical additives can also act as neurological time bombs, bioaccumulating slowly in the brain over a lifetime until Alzheimer's, Huntington's, and similar neurodegenerative diseases are triggered.

Within children's bodies and minds artificial flavorings and colorings can reach toxic levels much more quickly than in adults. A 2004 medical study published in *Archives of Disease in Childhood* examined four hundred children in Britain for signs of hyperactivity related to diet. Parents were asked to keep the children on a strict diet, free of all artificial preservatives and additives, for one month. Then for a week the children were given fruit drinks each day, laced with a cocktail of chemical additives—four colorings and one preservative—typical of what most children encounter with regularity.

"The observed effect of food additives and colorings in this community sample is substantial," concluded the medical team of researchers. Parents did daily ratings of their child's behaviors, and the results showed without equivocation that the additives affected their attention spans, moods, and ability to get along with others. One of the study authors, psychologist James Stevenson, said the study transformed his entire perspective on the relationship between food additives and the brain. "I'd worked in hyperactivity for a number of years and originally thought that diet was probably important only in an exceptional, odd group of children. Having done this work, I've changed my mind. Additives seem to be shifting behavior towards the more hyperactive end."

Other research has emerged linking processed foods to an alteration in brain chemistry that leads to addiction. In other words, a television ad that tells us "you can't eat just one" of those potato chips (or cookies or whatever) might be quite literally true. Ann Kelley, professor of neuroscience at the University of Wisconsin, has pioneered some of the research showing how common processed foods alter human brain chemistry in a way similar to drugs such as morphine, stimulating the release of pleasure chemicals in the brain that can result in cravings for specific foods.

MYTHS WE CHERISH

ARTIFICIAL SWEETENERS ARE SAFE

For many people the discovery of dangers associated with artificial sweeteners, those chemicals that trick our bodies into believing we have consumed sugar, will only arise as a consequence of personal suffering. Paula Baillie-Hamilton noticed how over time the diet sodas she was consuming altered her moods and gave her headaches. "I only stopped drinking diet drinks after hearing reports that not only had the artificial sweeteners in these drinks been shown to cause headaches and an agitated state like intoxication, exactly the symptoms I had previously experienced, but they had also been shown to cause brain, liver, lung, kidney, and lymphoreticular cancer."

Aspartame is the most common sweetening additive in more than one hundred diet and sugar-free products, ending up in soft drinks, cereals, frozen desserts, and tabletop sweeteners. It can also be found in such seemingly unlikely places as multivitamins, supplements, and pharmaceutical drugs. It contains three major components—methanol, phenylalanine, and aspartic acid. All three chemicals individually have been shown to either stimulate brain cells to death, upset hormone balances in the brain, or act as a nerve poison. The synergistic effects of these three chemical components on health are largely unknown.

The Canadian authors of *Hard To Swallow: The Truth About Food Additives* describe what happens when a diet drink containing aspartame is stored at a temperature of 85 degrees for a week or more: "There is no aspartame left in the soft drinks, just the components it breaks down into, like formaldehyde, formic acid, and diketopiperazine, a chemical which can cause brain tumours. All of these substances are known to be toxic to humans."

It took sixteen years for the FDA to finally approve the use of aspartame, because many of the animal studies testing its safety had produced a disturbing pattern of brain tumors. In 1980 an FDA Board of Inquiry voted unanimously against approving aspartame for human consumption. A year later the commissioner of the FDA, Arthur Hull Hayes Jr., overruled his agency's own scientists and approved aspartame for use in dry food products. He approved its use in carbonated beverages in 1983. Soon thereafter Hayes left the FDA and went to work for G.D. Searle & Company, the pharmaceutical company that manufactures aspartame. (Searle subsequently was bought by Monsanto, which was later sold to Pfizer.)

Over the next two years, after aspartame was added to soft drinks, Professor J. W. Olney of the Washington University in Saint Louis School of Medicine found that the incidence of brain cancer among U.S. citizens increased by 10 percent on average, representing about 1,500 new cases a year. For persons over age sixty-five, the increases in brain cancer rates were an astounding 60 percent or more. Olney was intrigued by the coincidence that studies of aspartame on lab animals had also found sharp increases in brain cancer, so he began conducting research and published a series of papers in *The New England Journal of Medicine* and elsewhere outlining how aspartame may cause brain damage in children.

Warnings about the toxicity of aspartame were issued in 1991 by the National Institutes of Health, which catalogued 167 adverse effects; in 1992 by the U.S. Air Force in a warning to its pilots not to fly after ingesting aspartame; and in 1994 by the United States Department of Health and Human Services, which detailed eighty-eight documented symptoms of aspartame toxicity. Here is a partial list of diseases thought to be exacerbated or triggered by this additive: birth defects, depression, mental retardation, chronic fatigue syndrome, brain tumors, epilepsy, multiple sclerosis, Parkinson's, and Alzheimer's.

Yet, this chemical toxin, once listed by the Pentagon as a prospective biochemical warfare weapon, remains widespread as an additive throughout the U.S. food supply and that of seventy other nations. It has been banned in Japan and a few other countries. What is the secret to its survival? British toxins expert Paula Baillie-Hamilton is blunt in her assessment. "Few incentives are as powerful as cold, hard cash." The manufacturers make so much money and exercise so much political influence, in her view, that the regulatory system has been manipulated and compromised.

Another reason aspartame survives is the fog of confusion caused by conflicting results from scientific studies of aspartame's health risks. Studies conducted by G.D. Searle, Monsanto, and other industry labs tend to declare aspartame safe, while studies conducted by independent scientists usually find it a danger to health. Ralph Walton, chairman of the Center for Behavioral Medicine at Northeastern Ohio University College of Medicine, did a comparative survey of these conflicting studies and found that eighty-three separate experiments over several decades—none funded by the aspartame industry—uncovered significant adverse health effects caused by the use of this synthetic sweetener.

Other artificial sweeteners introduced after aspartame do little to allay the health concerns about this class of synthetics. In 1988 the FDA approved acesulfame K, a synthetic two hundred times sweeter than sugar. It now appears in carbonated drinks, desserts, salad dressings, chewing gum, bakery mixes, and breath fresheners. In some experiments laboratory rats given acesulfame K have developed leukemia, tumors, and respiratory diseases. Aspartame is often combined with acesulfame K in products to mask bitterness, yet no studies are known to have been conducted on the synergistic effects in the body of combining these two additives.

A cruel irony underlying this saga is how these artificial sweeteners, commonly taken to lose weight, may actually become fat enhancers once absorbed by the human body. An American Cancer Association study tracking eighty thousand women for six years concluded, "Amongst women who gained weight, artificial sweetener users gained more than those who did not use the products." One reason may be that the synthetic chemicals affect hormone levels, thus undermining our own natural weight control systems by slowing metabolism and increasing appetite.

Using the FDA to suppress competition from natural sweetener alternatives to aspartame has been employed effectively to maintain market monopolies. A natural and virtually calorie-free sweetener and health remedy from South America, called stevia, fell into a bureaucratic black hole in 1994, when the FDA banned it, calling it "an unsafe food additive." This ban was enacted after a complaint was filed by a company the FDA refused to identify, charging that the stevia herb was being used in Celestial Seasonings tea without FDA approval.

Arizona congressman Jon Kyl charged that the FDA was engaging in "a restraint of trade to benefit the artificial-sweetener industry," and voiced suspicions the complaint had been filed by the makers of aspartame. Later, Congress passed legislation dealing with dietary supplements and allowed stevia to be sold as one such supplement, but in a strange twist, manufacturers were still prohibited from making any claims that even imply stevia is a sweetener. It is common knowledge that stevia is three hundred times sweeter than sugar, and without the calories, but broadcasting this truth in either labeling or advertising is considered a crime.

As for the FDA's continuing insistence that stevia "hasn't proven its safety as a food additive," we have only to examine the history of its use to see the transparency of that contention. Not only has there been hundreds of years of use among the people of South America, it has been used since the 1970s in Japan as a sweetener—and widely tested in Japanese laboratories—without any record of health complaints or concerns.

A journalist in 1997 requested that the FDA provide a list of all scientific studies the agency was using to justify its restrictions on the use of stevia. What the FDA provided on its short list is quite revealing. One of the scientists cited repeatedly by the FDA for having allegedly turned up findings that question stevia's safety is Mauro Alvarez, a researcher in Brazil. When Alvarez learned the FDA was using his research to justify restricting stevia, he released a public letter that was scathing: "The only possible way to report that my results showed detrimental effects is by taking information out of context." The objective of this misinformation, according to Alvarez, was "to keep the plant away from American consumers by attributing to it safety issues that do not exist. As a scientist with over fifteen years researching the safety of stevia and of many other plants used as food or food ingredients, I can assure that our conclusions in these various studies indicate that stevia is safe for human consumption."

MYTHS WE CHERISH

PET FOOD IS HARMLESS

After forty years treating health problems in pets, Richard Pitcairn has reached a conclusion that should sober every human with a pet in their lives. "Since I graduated from veterinary school in 1965, I've noticed a general deterioration in pet health. We now see very young animals with diseases that we used to see only in older animals. It is clear to me that an accumulation of poor health is being passed on from generation to generation; this accumulation increases with each step. Without the perspective of several decades, veterinarians just coming out of veterinary school think these degenerative conditions in younger animals are 'normal.' They do not realize what has happened over the passage of time. I believe that, along with poor quality nutrients, the *chemical additives* in pet food play a major part in that decline."

Many of us who have pet companions, particularly dogs and cats, have either seen firsthand or heard stories from other pet owners about how the animals contract illnesses, allergies, behavioral abnormalities, or diseases when consuming some commercial pet foods, only to miraculously recover once those processed foods are taken out of their diet. Given how pet foods are produced, we shouldn't be surprised.

Four of the five largest U.S. pet food companies are subsidiaries of major multinational corporations that also produce processed foods for humans. American pet owners spend an estimated $11 billion annually on animal foods made in part or whole from the scraps, rejects, and wastes—known as 4-D meat—collected and set aside by plants producing human food. This 4-D category stands for dead, diseased, dying, or disabled.

When these meats are rendered at rendering plants, they are often mixed with restaurant and supermarket refuse, euthanized animals from animal shelters, sawdust, cooking grease, and even roadkill, to create a concoction that is then laced with colorings, preservatives, fat stabilizers, and other chemical additives. The finished product is sold as dry food or, more often, as semimoist canned food (strangely enough, it also shows up as raw material for the cosmetics industry).

"Semimoist foods should be placed in a time capsule to serve as a record of modern technology gone mad," warns Alfred J. Plechner, in his book *Pet Allergies: Remedies For an Epidemic.* The preservatives in these foods, such as ethoxyquin, give them "a shelf life that spans eternity," and they bioaccumulate inside animals. Ethoxyquin has been detected in dogs' livers and tissues months after being removed from their diet and has been linked to cancer.

After rendering, the raw materials often receive other fat-stabilizer chemicals, BHA and BHT being the most common, to prevent rancidity. Both of these chemicals have been outlawed by many European countries because they are known to cause liver, brain, reproductive, and kidney problems. There is also evidence that the rendering process fails to remove sodium pentobarbital, the drug used to euthanize many animals that become pet food, and fails to destroy the hormones and antibiotics used to fatten livestock that is later rendered.

Other additives in moist food for pets have been identified by veterinarians as the source of additional health concerns. These additives include propylene glycol, used for texture and moisture; potassium sorbate, added as a preservative; propyl gallate, intended to retard spoilage; and sodium nitrite, used as a preservative and coloring agent. Several dyes added to pet food, such as Red No. 40 and Blue No. 2, make the food more visually appealing only to humans, since dogs and cats, not able to see colors the same way humans do, don't seem to care about the coloration of their food. Both of these colorings are also used in soft drinks and candies for humans, and each has been red-flagged by the Center for Science in the Public Interest as a possible danger to health.

As happens with human food, pet food processors use the term "artificial flavorings" as a convenient doorway through which to add unlabeled synthetic chemicals that have been called safe, though they have undergone little or no testing. Even when safety studies are done on additives and preservatives, only the direct toxicity is tested and not potential synergistic effects.

Anecdotal evidence continues to mount that synthetic chemical additives in food affect both humans and their pets in similar ways. A California woman was quoted in a 2004 issue of *Alternative Medicine* magazine making this comparison: "I have two children with disabilities. One has ADHD and the other suffers from depression. I took them to many doctors and not a single one ever asked me anything about what they eat. But when I took my dog to the vet to ask about his hyperactivity, the first question the vet asked was, 'What diet do you have him on?' It turns out something in his food was exacerbating his condition, and as soon as I switched him to a different formula, he greatly improved. Eventually I did a lot of nutritional interventions with both my kids, and they did much better as well."

MYTHS WE CHERISH

NASA HAS PERFECTED SYNTHETIC FOOD

A NASA classroom instructional guide for schoolchildren in 2001 posed these questions to teachers: "Can anything make kids covet fresh broccoli? Or yearn for lettuce straight from the garden?" The pamphlet answers with yes, just have your kids sample "the taste of dried, reconstituted vegetables" like those served to astronauts, then compare them to fresh vegetables. "Your students will gain a new perspective on the joy of greens."

After more than four decades of food experimentation and experience with sending humans into space, NASA still finds the task of trying to feed its astronauts a nutritious and palatable meal using synthetic ingredients to be an out-of-this-world challenge. While its food scientists may continue experimenting with new, exotic chemical formulas in attempts to mimic food nutrients for extended spaceflights, most NASA scientists have apparently resigned themselves to a "natural-is-better" approach.

Reducing weight and limiting the volume of materials stored in cabin space are priorities for every space mission. Those reasons alone would seem to make synthetic chemical foods more practical than heavier and bulkier natural foods. But NASA has instead opted for a strategy that will rely on growing natural crops in space to support astronaut survival and health.

In the early days of the space program astronauts ate synthetic and dehydrated foods from squeeze tubes. Ignorance about the nutritional needs of the human body reflected a desire to believe processed foods would be the future. A report during the late 1960s prepared by a scientist for the NASA Ames Research Center, for example, made this unsubstantiated claim about synthesizing food from pure chemicals: "It makes no difference to the body whether these substances come from a food of natural origin or are synthesized."

That sort of Frankenfood attitude about synthetic chemicals and the relationship of nutrition to health was largely abandoned by NASA when, as another food study later reported, "it quickly became apparent that these engineered foods were unacceptable in terms of odor, flavor, color, and texture." Synthetics failed to provide proper nutrition in comparison to salads and vegetables, which are considered the best possible sources for nutrients in space.

For trips to Mars and beyond, a leading candidate to become a bio-regenerative life support crop is quinoa, a weedlike food from the high Andes of South America, because of its high nutritional and mineral value. It also has the ability to remove carbon dioxide from the cabin atmosphere while generating food and water. Other high-nutrient crop candidates being considered for space harvesting include wheat, soybeans, lettuce, and white potatoes. Farming in space with as natural a group of ingredients as possible seems to be the future . . . or, maybe we should say it's back to the future!

What NASA has learned through trial and error, under the most severe conditions, the food processing industry chooses to ignore in its pursuit of convenience and profits from laboratory chemicals. As an illustration of NASA's wisdom in de-emphasizing spaceflight chemicals, a former senior science advisor to the American Institute for Cancer Research, T. Colin Campbell, drew this direct connection between the purity of the food we eat and our long-term prospects for health: "The vast majority of all cancers, cardiovascular diseases, and other forms of degenerative illness can be prevented simply by adopting a plant-based diet."

As we will explore in the next chapter, "disease industries" have sprung up in response to the health ravages of synthetic chemical foods, but what they offer as remedies for symptoms simply become additional toxic body burdens for us to bear.

TOXIC THREATS IN OUR FOOD

- Chemical flame-retardant residue (PBDEs) contaminate thirty-one of thirty-two common and name-brand grocery products, including fish, pork, turkey, chicken, cheese, butter, milk, eggs, and ice cream. Levels of PBDEs in the U.S. food supply are up to one hundred times higher than in any other country in the world because the U.S. use of this toxin in carpeting, electronics, and furniture is higher than anywhere else. The PBDEs bioaccumulate in the human body, and the long-term implications for health are unknown (from *Environmental Science & Technology*, 2004).

  Methyl bromide is a gas pesticide still used on tomatoes, strawberries, and other crops in the United States despite the U.S. government's having signed an international treaty banning most uses of the fumigant by 2005. The chemical harms the human neurological system. Growers of the affected crops complain that no effective and cheap replacement has been found for methyl bromide, so they have used their political influence to convince agencies of the U.S. government to grant them exemptions. Even golf courses have won this exemption (from Associated Press, "Despite treaty ban, U.S. farmers continue to use pesticide," November 27, 2005).

- Until 2002, plastics used to package foods were called "indirect food additives" by the FDA because it is generally understood that plastics leach chemicals into food, water, and the human body. But in that year the FDA changed the terminology to "food contact substances" so the public would not be unduly alarmed by the migration of plastics into food and water, especially bisphenol A (BPA) found in plastic water bottles. BPA is a well-known endocrine disrupter affecting development, memory, intelligence, and learning.

But duly alarmed is probably what we should be, if we listen to Victor O. Sheftel, chief environmental toxicologist at the Ministry of Health in Israel. He points out that the plastic called polymeric materials (PM) is used to package nearly 80 percent of our food. "The absence of acute poisonings with fatal outcome does not prove the safety of synthetic packaging materials. . . . It is well known that chronic effects may be observed as the result of repeated ingestion of a number of small doses, each in itself insufficient to cause an immediate acute reaction but in the long term having a cumulative toxic effect. Thus, PM and other widely used chemicals have introduced a problem of protracted action of low concentrations of chemicals upon human health."

- Of 9,282 people nationwide tested by the Centers for Disease Control and Prevention, 93 percent were found to have the insecticide TCP in their bodies and 99 percent carried a breakdown product of DDT. More than half of the test subjects had a dozen or more pesticides on average in their blood and urine. Much of this body burden had been absorbed through the foods they consumed.

- Commenting on the above statistics, a report by the Pesticide Action Network North America declared: "The human body is not designed to cope with synthetic pesticides. Yet we all carry a cocktail of chemicals designed to kill insects, weeds, and other agricultural and household pests. Many of the pesticides we carry in our bodies can cause cancer, disrupt our hormone systems, decrease fertility, cause birth defects, or weaken our immune systems. These are just some of the known detrimental effects of particular pesticides at very low levels of exposure. Almost nothing is known about the long-term impacts of multiple chemicals in the body over long periods" (from "Chemical Trespass," prepared by Pesticide Action Network North America, May 2004).

TOXIC THREATS IN OUR WATER

- A variety of consumer products used with tap water—such as some toothpastes, dishwashing liquids, and antimicrobial soaps—contain triclosan, a chemical that reacts with chlorinated water to produce chloroform gas, which is absorbed through a person's skin or inhaled. Chloroform can cause depression, liver problems, and cancer (from Virginia Tech University research, April 2005).
- Teflon-contaminated tap water is one reason 90 percent of Americans have Teflon residue in their blood. The highest levels of the Teflon chemical called C8 have been found accumulated in children six years old and under and in people over sixty years of age. Lab studies link C8 to a wide array of birth defects and developmental problems (from Edward Emmett, University of Pennsylvania research, August 2005).
- Drinking water for twenty million Americans is contaminated with a rocket fuel chemical called perchlorate—also used in fireworks, safety flares, and auto air bags—that persists in the environment and in the human body and can cause cancer and disrupt the thyroid gland. Even small disruptions of thyroid hormone levels during pregnancy can cause diminished intelligence, mental retardation, and impaired motor skills once the child is born (from Environmental Working Group study, 2005; and Environmental Protection Agency, 2002).
- Researchers at the University of Texas documented how taking showers and using dishwashers liberate trace amounts of chlorine and other chemicals from municipal water supplies into the air, and those trace chemicals are then inhaled and absorbed into the body. This process is known as stripping, and to avoid these released chemicals one would need to wear a gas mask when running the dishwasher or taking a shower (*The New York Times*, August 1, 2005).
- Municipal sewage treatment plants are not engineered to remove Pharmaceutical and Personal Care Product (PPCPs)

pollutants from the nation's water supply. When a United States Geological Survey report was issued in 2004 documenting how prescription drugs, steroids, antibiotics, pesticides, and other synthetic chemicals are being found at alarming levels everywhere during stream and groundwater testing, federal and state environmental officials made this revealing admission: Our nation's wastewater treatment plants are simply too unsophisticated to remove synthetic chemicals before water is recycled back into the environment. Nor can our municipal water treatment plants, despite the use of chlorine, neutralize all of these synthetic chemicals before we drink the tap water or bathe ourselves in it. Not only that, but most of the nation's soft drinks and beers are made with municipal tap water, which means we are slowly and cumulatively drugging ourselves in multiple ways.

CHAPTER FIVE

SORCERER'S APPRENTICES:
THE DRUG AND MEDICAL INDUSTRIES

". . . the whole imposing edifice of modern medicine, for all its breathtaking successes, is, like the celebrated Tower of Pisa, slightly off balance. It is frightening how dependent on drugs we are all becoming and how easy it is for doctors to prescribe them as the universal panaceas for our ills."

—Prince Charles, heir to the British throne

Western medicine's history of innovation is extremely short in comparison to the ancient medical traditions of India and China. The English word *drug* comes from the Dutch word *droog*, meaning "to dry," which was part of the process of turning plants into medicinal preparations. Patent medicines and the pharmaceutical industry evolved in relatively recent times from the lofty notion that combinations of secret ingredients could be cure-alls that protect the user from all manner of health woes.

Historical records indicate the first royal patent for a medicinal compound was granted by authorities in England during the early 1700s. By seeking a patent, the inventor agreed to reveal the ingredients of his medicine, so many cure-all creators opted instead to simply register their name brands, a tactic that helped to preserve the mystique they wove around their exotically named concoctions. By the 1750s more than two hundred medicines were protected by either patents or registration in England and its colonies.

America was the land of opportunity for patent medicine promoters during the nineteenth century as traveling medicine shows went from town to town, blending circuslike entertainment with slick marketing and promises of rejuvenated health. These health "lectures" from the backs of wagons later became drug commercials when radio emerged as a technological traveling road show. The cure-alls came to be generically known as "snake oil" and their promoters as "snake oil salesmen," because real snake oil, prized for its alleged curative qualities by various Indian tribes, was commonly sold in carnival sideshows to treat rheumatism, backaches, toothaches, and any other pain that needed relief.

The era of snake oil salesmen hit a big bump in the road of respectability in 1905 when *Collier's* magazine launched a series of articles exposing and attacking "The Great American Fraud" of patent medicine claims and deceptions. A direct consequence was the Pure Food and Drug Act passed by Congress, which took effect in 1906 and forced many cure-alls out of business or at least compelled them to change their advertising promises. But under this law the drug manufacturers and food processors were still not required to prove the safety of their products before offering them for sale. The burden was on government to prove the products unsafe before they could be ordered off the market.

Two developments in particular were instrumental in transforming the pharmaceutical industry into the all-embracing system it is today. In 1946 most U.S. drugmakers began commonly patenting instead of just registering individual drugs and their chemical ingredients, a practice that had previously been avoided to remain ethical in the eyes of consumers. Patenting of individual chemical molecule combinations gave drug manufacturers the ability to thwart competitors and to keep drug prices artificially high.

A second, equally important development came five years later when Congress passed a law requiring consumers to have prescriptions from physicians before they could purchase certain pharmaceutical drugs. This law created a marriage of convenience between the medical industry and the drug industry.

These developments in turn produced what has come to be known as "the magic bullet obsession." This is the idea—or myth—that by isolating chemical compounds down to the level of single molecules, the best possible healing agents, or bullets, can be found to treat illness and disease. While this may sometimes work in practice with new drugs during the short term, this fixation with single cures ignores all holistic and synergistic principles. In the long run we often experience higher medical costs and diminished health safety.

"All drugs go through the Cycle," a drug researcher told reporter Stephen Fried for his book, *Bitter Pills*. "First they're the silver bullet. Then they go into the trash. And then we come up with some mature reading of the thing. There's usually a category of patients for whom they are valuable. Unfortunately, we are very bad at deciding who is in that category."

One measurable impact of the emphasis on protecting molecular trade secrets in these magic bullets has been a proliferation of "me-too" drugs. "The great majority of 'new' drugs are not new at all but merely variations of older drugs already on the market," points out Marcia Angell, who monitored these trends while editor of *The New England Journal of Medicine*. Often new drugs represent nothing more than a change in a single molecule. In 2002, of seventy-eight drugs approved by the FDA, only seventeen contained any new active molecular ingredients, and only seven of these, conceded the FDA, actually were improvements over drugs already on the market.

Yet, in the face of these sobering statistics, we learn that the average elderly person in the United States takes more than one dozen prescription medications every single day. Prescription drug sales more than tripled in the United States between 1980 and 2000 to $200 billion annually, a figure representing half of all prescription drug sales in the entire world! In 2002, the combined profits of the ten largest U.S. drug companies were more than the combined profits of the other 490 corporations on the Fortune 500 list combined!

Using any drug as a magic bullet leaves "collateral damage" to our bodies, our health, and our personal wealth. Melvin Konner, in his pathbreaking book, *Medicine at the Crossroads*, describes some of the dangers of magic bullets this way: "More important than side effects, more important even than the evolution of resistance [to drug effectiveness] is an indirect result of the magic bullet viewpoint: the neglect of all the conditions that make life easy for the microbe, and that weaken the body's stance against invasion."

The conditions that make life easy for microbes, resulting in illness and disease, start with the weakening of the human immune system from improper nutrition and the body burden ravages of synthetic chemical toxins. Add to that mix the effects of synthetic drug over-prescription and dependence and we have a vicious cycle that fattens the drug and medical industries while depleting our own resources.

"Let the Un-Drugging of America Begin," read a cover story in a 2004 issue of *Forbes*, describing how the new enemy of the pharmaceutical industry is clean living. "Millions of us are popping prescription pills for innocuous ills when simple lifestyle changes of diet . . . are more effective and a lot cheaper. The results of pill dependence are insidious and devastating: billions of dollars in ever-higher drug costs; millions of people enduring sometimes highly toxic side-effects; and close to two million cases each year of drug complications that result in one hundred eighty thousand deaths or life-threatening illnesses."

What is the response of the pharmaceutical industry to these sorts of revelations? *Forbes* magazine summarized the industry's Alice in Wonderland attitude this way: "Big Pharma argues . . . that the real problem is undermedication." That's right, you read it correctly! The drug makers want us to believe that if only we ingest more of their synthetics the maladies that plague our culture will somehow seem less important or be forgotten, even if they don't really go away.

This attitude underscores an Achilles' heel of Big Pharma's entire synthetics belief system. They want us to believe that medicating symptoms is a good substitute for actually treating or curing the causes of illness and disease. If you have a migraine headache, do pharmaceutical drugs eliminate the cause? We all know the answer. All that pharmaceutical drugs do, for the most part, is to temporarily relieve symptoms in order to buy time in the hope that our own immune systems, if those systems aren't compromised, will kick into action and heal us.

NATURE'S GIFT ABUSED

A pattern I have noticed is that the more synthetic a drug turns out to be, the more toxic its potential effects on the human body, especially on the immune system. By way of comparison, consider the relative toxicity of illegal drugs. Of the four most common illegal drugs in use today— marijuana, cocaine, heroin, and methamphetamine—the most synthetic of the four and simultaneously the most addictive and toxic to health is methamphetamine.

Marijuana is the closest to nature of the four and not coincidentally the least injurious to health. While it can be habit-forming, there is little evidence that it is physically addictive. Synthetic processes extract cocaine from the naturally occurring coca plant, and heroin from the naturally occurring poppy plant. But with methamphetamine both the process of extraction and the chemicals comprising the drug itself are all synthetic.

The documented health impacts of meth use are wide-ranging and severe: destruction of brain cells responsible for memory and emotion, seizures, infections, tooth loss, and gum disease. People high on meth are subject to uncontrollable bursts of anger in response to what might otherwise be normal irritations. During the early 1990s I researched and wrote an article for *Reader's Digest* about an epidemic of infant murders in the high desert of Southern California committed by people intoxicated on meth. I had the unpleasant experience of standing in a hospital intensive care ward with sheriff's deputies when the life support system was turned off on a brain-dead eight-month-old girl, whose mother's meth-addicted boyfriend had shaken into a coma.

Nature's gift to us is our immune system, a highly specialized frontline defense against illness and disease that insures our health as naturally occurring from birth. The ancient Greek physician Hippocrates, considered to be the father of Western medicine, may not have known with certainty that the human immune system existed, but he knew intuitively as evidenced by his statement, "The natural healing force within each of us is the greatest force in getting well."

Synthetic chemicals, whether legal or illegal, can damage our immune systems in two ways, either suppressing it or over-stimulating it. Suppression can create conditions for illnesses like the flu or diseases like cancer, while over-stimulation can cause allergic reactions and auto-immune system disorders.

Many of us after a stressful period in our lives have come down with colds or other ailments, so we know firsthand the impact that stress can have on our immune systems. Even more devastating to immunity is what can happen in the wake of tragedy, such as the death of a spouse. Combine life's stresses with the body burden of stresses foisted on us by synthetic chemical exposure, combined again with nutritional deficiencies and overuse of prescription drugs, and we have a formula for immune system breakdown and chronic ill health.

Our culture treats medical emergencies and the symptoms of illness and disease relatively well in the short term, thanks to remarkable technological advances in medical science. We are mostly failures, however, when it comes to the prevention of illness and disease and in understanding the importance of using diet to enhance the strength of our immune systems.

"During medical consultations, the concept that chemical exposure may have contributed in some way to a patient's problem doesn't even enter the doctor's head," observes physician and toxins expert Paula Baillie-Hamilton. "Doctors are trained to believe chemicals, i.e. drugs, are the answer, not the problem."

Perhaps modern medicine's drug dependence will one day be viewed as just another of its faddish fixations and blind oversights. Three historical examples provide cause for hope in that regard and illustrate how a change in perspective, even for as hallowed a profession as medicine, often only comes about through the humiliations of experience.

Just a half century ago *The Journal of the American Medical Association*, as well as state medical journals, published advertising from tobacco manufacturers, my favorite being the Chesterfield cigarette ad that reassured doctors that "cigarettes are just as pure as the water you drink." Then there were the Camel cigarette ads that touted this brand as the one "more doctors smoke than any other cigarette." When the surgeon general's report in 1964 condemned smoking as bad for health, the AMA refused to endorse this plea to stop smoking and instead accepted $18 million more from tobacco companies over the ensuing nine years. Eventually common sense and the weight of scientific evidence prevailed to change the AMA's position about the dangers of cigarette smoking.

A second faddish belief that now seems absolutely barbaric in its insensitivity was the conviction promoted by the medical industry that children experience pain less severely than adults. Infants underwent major surgery without anesthetics right through the 1960s, on the theory infants wouldn't retain a memory of their trauma. Finally, after untold thousands of traumas being committed, research proved that youngsters actually experience pain *more* intensely than adults do.

Next on my hit parade of medical fads is one that gripped the medical profession for decades and almost ensnared me as a child. My tonsils would swell and redden every time I came down with a cold, and doctors urged my mother to put me in the hospital for a tonsillectomy. Surgical removal of tonsils was considered appropriate for most any child during the 1950s and 1960s because physicians viewed the tonsils as nothing more than a bacteria-collecting nuisance.

Fortunately for me, my mother had the good intuitive sense to resist these "let's cut him up" entreaties, and as I got older, my tonsils never got infected again. By the early 1970s these surgeries almost disappeared as physicians realized that tonsil irritation was just something that most children outgrow. "A decades-long surgical fad swept up millions of American children in its overenthusiasm," remembers Dr. Melvin Konner. "Today tonsillectomies are done on only a small fraction of children."

MYTHS WE CHERISH

THE GOVERNMENT INSURES THAT DRUGS ARE SAFE

During the first few years of the twenty-first century, four authoritative books appeared, each written by a physician turned medical school academic, demolishing some of our fondest myths about the pharmaceutical industry and the true nature of its symbiotic relationship to modern Western medicine. Three of the physicians—Marcia Angell, Jerry Avorn, and John Abramson—are associated with Harvard Medical School, while the fourth, Jay S. Cohen, serves as a professor of medicine at the University of California at San Diego.

What these medical authorities share is a conclusion that modern medicine's dependence on synthetic chemicals manufactured by pharmaceutical companies often results in a failure to adequately protect public health. That failure begins with the relationship that evolved over the past century between the FDA and the drugmakers this agency has been tasked to regulate.

"There is a comforting shared myth that by the time the FDA approves a new drug, the product has been studied exhaustively and determined to be a worthwhile new addition, and that all its actions in the body, both good and bad, are well defined," writes Avorn in his book, *Powerful Medicines*. "In fact none of these assumptions is quite correct. The FDA itself does not study any drugs prior to approval, relying on the company that makes the product to generate that information."

Our government depends on safety data supplied by the drug manufacturers to make its approval decisions. To Angell, former editor in chief of *The New England Journal of Medicine*, relying on the drug companies "for unbiased evaluations of their products makes about as much sense as relying on beer companies to teach us about alcoholism."

While we might hope and pray that medical tests of drug safety by pharmaceutical companies are conducted without distortion by the profit motive or competitive pressures, especially since so many lives are at stake, Abramson and Angell both suggest that widespread patterns of deception occur in these drug trials. Rigged medical studies, misrepresented research results, and "the propagandizing of physicians and the public by manipulative pharmaceutical companies," writes Abramson in his book, *Overdo$ed,* "creates a corruption of medical science." Angell is no less candid in her own book, *The Truth About the Drug Companies*: "Is there some way companies can rig clinical trials to make their drugs look better than they are? Unfortunately, the answer is yes. Trials can be rigged in a dozen ways and it happens all the time."

A possible case in point occurred in late 2005 as a new diabetes drug headed to the marketplace, having had its safety endorsed by an FDA panel. Two prominent Ohio cardiologists did an independent analysis of the testing data for this drug and rushed their findings onto a Web site maintained by *The Journal of the American Medical Association* "to head off a Vioxx-like fiasco, a public health catastrophe." They had discovered that this treatment for type 2 diabetes called muraglitazar, developed by Bristol-Myers Squibb and Merck & Company, causes many more instances of death from heart attacks and strokes than company test data had portrayed to the FDA. The two Cleveland cardiologists uncovered a pattern of omissions in data presented to the FDA that created an unwarranted "illusion of safety." *JAMA*'s editor in chief, Catherine DeAngelis, was scathing in her description of the FDA's oversight failure: "It is beyond me why individuals who are supposed to be overseeing the safety of the public would take a chance [with public health] when it's not necessary."

If the system fails the only effective way to judge drug safety or drug dangers is by the health effects reported among those unknowing human guinea pigs who are the first consumers of new prescription drugs. Since 1997, reported toxic health effects have resulted in the withdrawal of more drugs from the marketplace than ever before in history. Four of those withdrawn—Redux, Rezulin, Propulsid, and Seldane—were prescribed to nearly twenty million people before the toxic effects began showing up.

The human costs of this ongoing experiment with drug safety have become staggeringly large. At least 106,000 people die each year just in hospitals from drug side effects, according to a study in 1998 by *The Journal of the American Medical Association*. That averages out to around 300 deaths a day, every day, from legal toxic drugs.

In his book *Over Dose*, Cohen quotes a study by three university professors in *The Journal of the American Medical Association* that determined that at least 51 percent of all FDA-approved drugs "have serious adverse effects not detected prior to approval." This revelation prompted Cohen to indignantly write: "Think about this: More than half of our drugs, after being deemed 'safe' by the FDA and then prescribed to millions of people, are subsequently detected to have previously unrecognized, medically serious side effects. No wonder we have a side-effect epidemic."

An investigation by *Consumer Reports* (January 2006) examined a dozen common types of prescription drugs sold in 140 brand-name or generic versions and found a range of adverse side effects including stroke, heart attack, and kidney failure. In every case these side effects "were undetected or underestimated when the FDA approved them for use."

Blame for this "illusion of safety" was laid equally on the drug manufacturers and the FDA. "Some companies have withheld publication of studies that found serious risks, or have failed to conduct post-approval studies that they promised," charged the magazine. For its part the FDA "lacks the power to compel companies to complete studies after drug approval, force doctors to report adverse reactions, or dictate new warning labels."

Commenting on the public perceptions of objectivity and safety afforded by the FDA, an FDA commissioner, Herbert Lay, made this revealing statement in 1969, which still holds true today: "The thing that bugs me is that people think the FDA is protecting them. It isn't. What the FDA is doing and what the public thinks it's doing are as different as night and day."

MYTHS WE CHERISH

ONE DOSE FITS ALL

When you see a physician and receive a prescription for a drug, the odds are high you will get a "one dose size fits all" sort of treatment. Most of us never give a second thought to how this common practice defies common sense.

Every drug company seems to believe that synthetic drugs targeting specific maladies can work in the same way for everyone. This idea is marketed to physicians and consumers and has dangerous repercussions: it encourages physicians to prescribe higher drug doses than are necessary; it ignores individual metabolic variations; and it creates a synergy in which more toxic drugs are prescribed in attempts to reduce the side effects of other medications.

Individual variation in how we absorb and metabolize any prescribed drug, or any synthetic chemical for that matter, can extend from a 400 percent to even a 4,000 percent difference in the dosage required between one person and another, according to the American Medical Association. But drug manufacturers try to standardize, almost without exception, every prescription drug, and most physicians usually play along in this game despite the threat to their patients' health.

The former director of the FDA's Center for Drug Evaluation and Research, Carl Peck, was quoted by *The New York Times* in 1999 as charging that "one dose fits all is a marketing myth, but it's the holy grail that every drug company tries to achieve."

Physicians want maximum effectiveness from the drugs they prescribe, and higher doses produce this maximum effect. Since physicians and not patients are choosing which drugs are used, prescription drugs are automatically tailored to the preferences expressed by these medical practitioners.

The result can be disastrous for those of us being treated as guinea pigs of convenience. Jay Cohen saw these repercussions firsthand in connection with Prozac, the widely used antidepressant. "I understand why so many of my patients reacted adversely to Prozac. They were getting overmedicated. They were getting doses 100 to 400 percent greater than some of them needed."

In one study, 30 percent of people on Prozac quit after experiencing side effects. *The Journal of Clinical Psychiatry* reported that 85 percent of Prozac users suffered diarrhea, 70 percent experienced profuse sweating, and 50 percent gained weight. Despite these and other reported side effects, Prozac's manufacturer, Eli Lily, continued recommending that doctors prescribe 20 milligrams or more as the starting dose.

"So when a patient develops a side effect, rather than simply reducing the dose without any extra cost to anyone," reports Cohen in *Over Dose*, "doctors do what they know best—write another prescription. Very few physicians go to the trouble of adjusting drug dosages to fit their patients. Most don't deviate from the drug companies' recommendations. They don't individualize."

Antibiotics are another category of overprescribed "one dose fits all" drugs whose abuse negatively affects us both as individuals and as a society. Ninety percent of the sore throats we Americans experience each year are viral in nature and immune to antibiotics, but medical statistics indicate that 73 percent of the estimated 6.7 million visits by adults to physicians complaining of a sore throat between 1989 and 1999 resulted in a prescription for antibiotics.

That means many if not most prescriptions written for antibiotics are inappropriate, which seems like an overly polite way of describing this gigantic scam. Physicians argue they are only responding to the demands of patients who want antibiotics prescribed whether they are appropriate to the illness or not. It may even be that antibiotics are effective indirectly and unintentionally by activating the placebo response in people, that "mind over matter" potential we all have for self-healing.

There are two big problems with the antibiotics racket: it is now the leading cause of adverse drug reactions in the United States and it produces resistant strains of deadly bacteria. Every body of water in the nation, including drinking water, tested for drug residues turns up antibiotics that have accumulated from human waste and from runoff traceable to animal farms that overuse antibiotics as growth promoters. These residues bioaccumulate in fish and other aquatic life to provide us with still another jolt of antibiotics somewhere else along the food consumption chain.

We are disrupting our body's inner ecology by killing off harmless bacteria that may protect our health by bolstering our immune systems. *Discover* magazine featured an appropriately titled article, "Are Antibiotics Killing Us?" in its October 2005 edition that made an irrefutable case showing how antibiotics use has "accelerated the spread of drug-resistant genes to the public" and this threatens our very survival.

Between 2000 and 2003 the reported cases of a bacterial infection known as C.diff doubled in U.S. hospitals. Other similar outbreaks were documented in Canada, England, and the Netherlands. This dangerous strain had quickly mutated to resist standard antibiotics treatments and began infecting young people for the first time, causing many severe illnesses and fatalities. An article in the December 21, 2005 issue of *The Journal of the American Medical Association* reported that persons taking Prilosec and Prevacid, both popular heartburn medications, were three times more likely to be diagnosed with C.diff as those not taking the medication. Apparently a type of synergy had developed between the overuse of antibiotics and the use of heartburn medications to create an intestinal environment conducive to the spread of this meaner and nastier strain of bacteria.

"Every time we take a course of penicillin or erythromycin we don't need, we turn our own bodies into little laboratories for the breeding of resistant germs," Melvin Konner warns us. "Widespread feeding of antibiotics to livestock exacerbates the problem. And the more resistance there is, the more money pharmaceutical companies have to invest in new antibiotic research, money that they then feel they have to recoup—as well as gaining substantial profit—by charging very high prices for the very newest drugs."

MYTHS WE CHERISH

FLUORIDATED WATER IS HEALTHY FOR US

One of the more memorable and hilarious scenes in the early 1960s satirical movie *Dr. Strangelove* featured a monologue by a U.S. military general ranting and raving about the necessity to protect "our precious bodily fluids" from contamination by fluoride in drinking water, presumably because the drug had been placed there as part of a Communist plot to control the world.

Ridiculing people who feared the health effects of fluoridated water by labeling them a lunatic fringe proved extraordinarily effective for many decades in protecting fluoride from serious scrutiny. After all, we were constantly being assured by authority figures in medicine, government, and industry that consuming fluoride was not only safe, it would help to ensure that we maintained good dental health. Who could argue with that?

About 66 percent of public municipal water systems in the United States serving 170 million people had been fluoridated by the dawn of the twenty-first century, yet most of the countries in Western Europe—from France and Germany to Italy and Switzerland—continue to reject adding fluoride to their drinking water. Did they know something we refuse to accept?

It might be useful to recall how fluoridation came about in the first place. A scientist working under a grant from the Aluminum Company of America made the initial public proposal in 1939 to add fluoride to public water supplies in the belief that it would help prevent tooth decay. In 1945 the first barrels of sodium fluoride were added to the drinking water in Grand Rapids, Michigan. When the United States Public Health Service endorsed fluoridation a few years later, many cities and entire states quickly followed that advice.

There was an ulterior motive for the aluminum industry and the fertilizer industry to promote the fluoridation idea. A by-product of factory smokestacks operated by both industries was a toxic waste called silicofluoride that contained lead, cadmium, arsenic, and other toxins. Instead of these industries having to pay for the disposal of this waste (today at an estimated cost of $8,000 a truckload), fluoridation enabled both to make money by selling the waste for use in public water supplies.

Using public water as a vehicle to deliver a drug—and one that is among the most toxic substances on the planet, used as an active ingredient in many pesticides—was an idea that concerned some physicians and scientists at the time. It even initially drew opposition from the dental profession. A 1944 editorial in *The Journal of the American Dental Association* warned that water fluoridation's prospects for harming human health "far outweigh those for the good."

Once dentists came aboard the fluoridation bandwagon along with public health–minded politicians, and with backing from a public relations campaign funded by aluminum and fertilizer industry coffers, there was no stopping the fluoridation juggernaut. Industry-funded studies began to appear in dental and medical journals showing improvements in dental health apparently resulting from fluoridated water, and that was all the proof most people needed to accept fluoridation's benefits as the gospel truth. Anyone who disagreed was branded a right-wing nut.

Periodically a courageous voice with impeccable scientific credentials spoke up to sound an alarm about fluoridation's potential dangers, only to be dismissed as eccentric. In 1975, for instance, the chief chemist emeritus of the National Cancer Institute, Dean Burk, declared that fluoride in water "causes more human cancer, and causes it faster, than any other chemical."

Two years later some members of Congress inquired about whether federal health authorities, after a quarter-century of experience with fluoridation, had ever tested fluoridated water as a cause of cancer. The answer was no. More than a decade passed before these tests were finally performed. The results caused a brief uproar. Young male rats exposed to fluoridated water developed both bone cancer and liver cancer.

These results were quickly attacked on a variety of grounds—flawed methodology, incomplete results, animal studies aren't always reliable, etc.—and then ignored by the fluoridation establishment. But other researchers, emboldened by the precedent this study set, began conducting their own experiments into fluoride's effects on health. In 1992, three U.S. scientists found evidence of Alzheimer's-like symptoms in laboratory animals exposed to fluoridated water that had apparently carried traces of aluminum into the animals' brains. That same year a study appeared in *The Journal of the American Medical Association* connecting water fluoridation to an increased risk of hip fractures.

The negative studies about fluoride's effects on health built into a tsunami during the 1990s. Here are just a few examples: the medical journal *Neurotoxicology and Teratology* found evidence that fluoride accumulates in the human body and creates motor-skills dysfunction and learning disabilities; two separate studies in the journal *Fluoride* showed that in areas where water supplies were fluoridated, children's IQs were lower than normal. Other science papers in *Fluoride* drew connections between the chemical and thyroid abnormalities, arthritis, even Down's syndrome in children.

Even the argument that put fluoride into drinking water in the first place—that it prevents tooth decay—came under a sustained challenge. A study in 1995 by the California Department of Health Services revealed that money spent on dental work actually increased in areas where water was fluoridated in that state, while dental costs declined in communities without fluoridated water. In the July 2000 issue of *The Journal of the American Dental Association*, John D. B. Featherstone of the University of California at San Francisco, concluded that ingesting fluoride from tap water does little to prevent tooth decay. Fluoride only works when directly applied to teeth in the form of toothpaste.

By 2004, an estimated five hundred peer-reviewed scientific studies had appeared indicating health problems associated with fluoride consumption. Rather than accept the possibility that water fluoridation may be a flawed idea, fluoride's proponents have continued reacting with a sort of *Dr. Strangelove* logic that relies upon dismissive ridicule. A statement posted on the Web site of the American Council on Science and Health, a group financed in part by the chemical industry, called criticisms of water fluoridation "a fake controversy" that "represents one of the major triumphs of quackery over science in our generation."

Undaunted by these charges, a prominent Canadian dental expert, Hardy Limeback, head of the Department of Preventive Dentistry at the University of Toronto, publicly apologized in 1999 for having been a proponent of water fluoridation. "Because of the cumulative properties of the toxins, the detrimental effects on human health are catastrophic." He pointed out that in Toronto, after thirty-six years of fluoridating water, the cavity rate was higher than in Vancouver, which had never fluoridated its water supply. For a half century the well-intentioned dental profession foisted misinformation about fluoride onto an unsuspecting public, claims Limeback, and the result has been "a poisoning of our children."

It is these cumulative effects of fluoride in our bodies that should most concern us. A United States Department of Health and Human Services report has estimated that the average person absorbs about seven parts per million of fluoride a day from all sources combined—water, food, air, even from pesticides that contain fluoride. By contrast, the optimal level of exposure to fluoride, according to the EPA, should be no more than *one* part per million a day, but public water supplies use standards of no more than four parts per million. By contrast, the World Health Organization set a fluoride-safety standard of just 1.5 parts per million.

This discrepancy between what we absorb and the levels at which fluoride is safe, along with government studies showing fluoridated water to be instrumental in causing chronic fatigue and fibromyalgia, so alarmed EPA scientists that their union, representing 1,500 civil servants, called for a moratorium on fluoridation. "Like most Americans, including many physicians and dentists, most of our members had thought that fluoride's only effects were beneficial. . . . We too believed assurances of safety," read the statement by J. William Hirzy, Senior Vice President of chapter 280 of the National Treasury Employees Union in May 1999. "Since then our opposition to drinking water fluoridation has grown, based on the scientific literature."

Hirzy summed up the loony logic of injecting fluoride toxic wastes into our drinking water: "If this stuff gets out into the air, it's a pollutant.

If it gets into the river, it's a pollutant. If it gets into the lake, it's a pollutant. But if it goes right straight into your drinking water system, it's not a pollutant. That's amazing!"

In late 2005 the Centers for Disease Control and Prevention released a report disclosing that 60 percent of children from ages six to nineteen have never had a cavity in their permanent teeth. Less than 35 percent of children could make that claim in 1980. Once again the CDC's statistical journal, *Morbidity and Mortality Weekly Report,* used these statistics as an opportunity to trot out its contention that fluoridation is one of the nation's ten great public health achievements. If you read the CDC report carefully, however, a huge Achilles' heel in this argument becomes apparent. An exception to these findings about the overall decline in cavities is poor children. Guess who drinks larger volumes of tap water containing fluoride than the children from middle-class and wealthy families, who can afford unfluoridated bottled spring water? It is children from lower-income groups. This irony was apparently lost on the CDC.

A sea change in attitudes about the safety of adding fluoride to water seems to be under way in the United States. A major article on the growing opposition to fluoridation appeared in *Time* magazine (October 24, 2005) and described how tooth decay "has plummeted even in regions where there is little or no fluoride in the water," and warned that "fluoride is indisputably toxic; it was once commonly used in rat poison." The article revealed that a Harvard University study had been suppressed because it "showed a sevenfold increased risk of osteosarcoma in preadolescent boys from fluoridated water." Furthermore, "in Western Europe, where the drop in tooth decay in recent decades is as sharp as that in the U.S., seventeen of twenty-one countries have either refused or discontinued fluoridation" because of health safety concerns.

MYTHS WE CHERISH

WE GET ALL THE VITAMINS WE NEED

If we define a drug as any chemical that influences the functioning of the human body, vitamins and minerals are drugs in the same category as other pharmaceuticals. The difference is that we require a daily absorption of vitamins, mostly through our food, throughout our life if we are to stay healthy. In that sense vitamins are the most important drugs we will ever use, and as with other types of medicine, we have a choice between natural and synthetic.

Over the past half century we have been subjected to a series of contradictory messages about the proper level of vitamins and nutrients in our food. These mixed messages come from the food, drug, and medical industries, and the regulatory agencies of the government.

The first message given us was "you get all of the vitamins and minerals you need from the food you eat." When nutritional research cast doubt on that claim, we were told to "take multivitamin supplements and your nutrient needs will be met." Now we seem to have come full circle again. Food processors have been adding synthetic vitamins to create "functional foods," and we are once again being assured we can get all of the nutrients we need from the food we eat.

For an illustration of this conflict look at what happened with the reputation of vitamin E. In a 1971 official statement, the FDA discouraged supplementation with this claim: "Vitamin E displays no known medical therapeutic effects." By 1990 the agency had done a complete reversal and touted vitamin E as an essential nutrient that is capable of preventing oxidation of polyunsaturated fatty acids in the body, which would lead to cell damage.

"Federal bureaucrats generally have been skeptical about the need for supplements or the existence of nutritional problems," say pharmacologist Joe Graedon and medical anthropologist Teresa Graedon, authors of *Dangerous Drug Interactions*. "Unless people start developing classic deficiency diseases such as scurvy, pellagra, or beriberi, no one is likely to worry."

But we do have cause for concern. "It is a myth that we get all the vitamins we need in our daily diets," insists Anthony Verlangieri, director of a research lab at the University of Mississippi School of Pharmacy.

Our foods lose essential nutrients at every step of the process from their growth to our dining tables. It starts with the nutrient-depleted soils in which the crops are grown, then the loss accelerates during food shipping, processing, storage, and finally cooking.

Nutrition scientist Shari Lieberman, co-author of *The Real Vitamin & Mineral Book*, cautions that "even if we ate a 'balanced' diet, our food has less nutrition to begin with because it is raised using synthetic chemicals, and then it is stored and processed to within an inch of its life. The flour used to make white bread has been depleted of over twenty nutrients, including up to 40 percent of vitamin C, 85 percent of vitamin B_6, and 72 percent of zinc. The manufacturers then put back a handful of these nutrients (five, to be exact) and call the result 'enriched.' "

Because vitamin E causes food to turn rancid sooner, food processors remove it to extend the shelf life of food products. With wheat grain, about 86 percent of vitamin E is lost anyway during milling and processing into white bread. One theory holds that heart disease went from a few reported cases in the early twentieth century to being a major killer at the end of that century as a consequence of vitamin E being stripped from our food.

A scientific nail in the coffin of the "we get all the supplements we need in food" myth came in 2002 when *The Journal of the American Medical Association* published an article that reviewed thirty years of medical research about the relationship between vitamins and chronic diseases. The trend was clear, showing that most people get less-than-optimal intakes of vitamins from food, and that puts them at increased risk for cardiovascular disease, cancer, and other ailments. "All adults should take one multivitamin daily," the two Harvard researchers concluded.

But all multivitamins aren't created equal. We have indoctrinated ourselves, based on drug industry advertising, to believe our bodies do not know the difference between vitamins synthesized in a laboratory and the vitamins that occur naturally in fruits and vegetables.

You will find three types of vitamins sold today: the naturally occurring (taken directly from plant or fruit sources), the much more numerous brands of synthetic, and the equally numerous yeast tablets injected with synthetic chemicals. This latter category misleads the consuming public because, even though these synthetics are labeled as natural under FDA guidelines (and only because they include yeast), they are still synthetic imitations. Both categories of vitamin synthetics are "magic bullets" developed by the pharmaceutical industry.

Soon after a Swiss chemist succeeded in artificially synthesizing vitamin C in 1933, the drugmaker Hoffman-LaRoche manufactured the first synthetic vitamins and an industry was born. Thirteen vitamins in all would eventually be discovered and industrially synthesized in laboratories: four are fat soluble, meaning they can be stored in the body (vitamins A, D, E, and K), while the other nine are water soluble, meaning they cannot be stored and must be consumed frequently (vitamin C and the eight B vitamins.)

Today the vitamin industry is dominated by six pharmaceutical companies that produce about 97 percent of all raw materials for the synthetic vitamins we find on store shelves. Their vitamins are made from coal tars and use artificial colorings, preservatives, disintegrents, coating materials, and other additives.

Synthetic vitamin C is really just ascorbic acid, comparable to the outer skin of an orange; 90 percent of the ascorbic acid in the United States is manufactured at a facility in Nutley, New Jersey, owned by Roche. In this plant the ascorbic acid is derived from cornstarch, corn sugar, and volatile acids mixed in a fermentation process. Most U.S. vitamin companies purchase this ascorbic acid, bottle it, and attach their own labels before selling it as vitamin C. Even less well known, most synthetic vitamin E comes from an Eastman Kodak plant, where it is a by-product of an emulsification process used to manufacture film. After purification it is sold to the supplements industry.

At the level of molecules seen under an electron microscope, synthetic and natural vitamins may look similar to some chemists, but they don't assimilate the same way in the human body. Studies of both vitamin C and vitamin E show that the naturally occurring forms are more absorbable by the body and more biologically active than synthetics.

The science studies demonstrating the superiority of naturally occurring vitamins over synthetics have been published in such journals as *Annals of the New York Academy of Sciences*, *The American Journal of Clinical Nutrition*, and Britain's *Royal Society of Chemistry*. In a 1998 study at Oregon State University six volunteers were given 150-milligram doses of synthetic vitamin E and later the same dose of vitamin E from natural sources. Urine tests showed conclusively that the human body prefers natural vitamin E by its retention of it and by how quickly it excretes the synthetic version. Robert Acuff, director of the Center for Nutrition Research at

East Tennessee State University, did a review of thirty published studies on the differences between natural and synthetic vitamin E and concluded that the natural form delivers twice the health benefits of synthetics because it is the one our bodies were designed to use.

Newspaper headlines in late 2004 trumpeted the news of a study published by *Annals of Internal Medicine* that found taking vitamin E supplements fails to prevent heart disease. A friend of mine in the vitamin industry pointed out that this study, like nearly every other health-related study of vitamins, used synthetic and not natural sources. Even the news coverage of this negative study indirectly alluded to such a bias. "Studies also show that healthy people who eat vitamin-rich food seem to have less heart disease," read the Associated Press report. "Experts say that perhaps antioxidants [such as vitamin E] work when only in food."

Naturally occurring substances seem to contain a "lifeforce" that synthetics cannot duplicate. That lifeforce is a product of synergy, and synthetics lack the capacity to induce natural synergies. With any vitamin there is an accompanying x-factor of supporting compounds, without which the beneficial effects on the body are diminished. Nobel Prize laureate Albert Szent-Györgyi was one of the first to notice how scurvy, a disease caused by vitamin C deficiency, could never be cured by the ascorbic acid component of vitamin C alone but required the complete matrix of vitamin C components found in food.

A friend of mine, Scott Treadway, has spent thirty years as an expert on vitamin formulation and draws a clear distinction between synthetic and natural. "Although we have been led to believe that ascorbic acid, a synthesized form of vitamin C, is really vitamin C, *it is not*. Alpha tocopherol is not vitamin E. Retinoic acid is not vitamin A. And so on through the other vitamins. Vast energy and resources have been expended to make these myths part of conventional wisdom. However, the truth is that vitamins are not individual molecular compounds. Vitamins are biological complexes. In addition to ascorbic acid, real vitamin C must include bioflavonoids [the natural pigments in fruits and vegetables] like hesperidin, rutin, quercetin, tannins, along with other naturally occurring compounds. Mineral cofactors must be available in proper amounts. If any of these parts are missing, there is no vitamin activity."

A pioneer in drawing such distinctions was Royal Lee, who wrote in a 1956 issue of the medical journal *Applied Trophology* that a natural vitamin is "a working process consisting of the nutrient, enzymes, coenzymes, antioxidants, and trace mineral activators."

Since then some chemists have noted that at the molecular level there is a difference between natural molecules and the synthetic ones designed to mimic them. Two Canadian chemists writing in an American Chemical Society journal in 2002 observed that "it is common knowledge in medicinal chemistry" that synthetic molecules "generally lead to a less specific and weaker activity" than natural molecules. Additionally, "the process of producing synthetic analogues radically alters the numbers and ratios of different atom types," resulting in less bioavailability.

What the pharmaceutical industry today foists upon us as vitamins essential to our health are actually more of the synthetic "magic bullet" drugs that our bodies treat as toxins, that have weakened our immune systems, that contaminate our foods, and that manipulate our health hopes and our fears.

MYTHS WE CHERISH

VACCINATIONS ARE ALWAYS BENEFICIAL

According to most public health specialists today, the important advances against infectious diseases in the late nineteenth and early twentieth centuries came about not from the introduction of vaccines, but from improved public health resulting from cleaner water and more effective sewage disposal.

Vaccines have proven most beneficial as an emergency medical treatment when epidemics rage out of control. For instance, in 1988 about 350,000 people, mostly in West Africa, lost their eyesight from river blindness caused by a black fly–carried parasite. The drug company Merck produced a drug called ivermectin to cure this scourge, and it was distributed by the World Health Organization to affected countries, virtually eliminating this contagion.

But vaccines aren't always safe or effective. Here are four examples:

- A medical journal, *The Lancet,* reported in 1980 that a vaccine trial in India involving 260,000 people discovered that more cases of tuberculosis had occurred in people vaccinated against TB than among the unvaccinated.

- *The Journal of the American Medical Association* printed an article on measles in 1990 that revealed: Although more than 95 percent of school-aged children in the U.S. are vaccinated against measles, measles outbreaks continue to occur in schools, and most cases in this setting occur among previously vaccinated children.

- Though from 1990 through 1993 the FDA counted 54,072 adverse reactions to vaccinations, the agency also admitted this total represented only about 10 percent of actual adverse reactions because most physicians were reluctant to report the problems.

- In a 1994 issue of *The New England Journal of Medicine* it was reported that at least 80 percent of children under the age of five who came down with whooping cough had been vaccinated against whooping cough.

There is another downside to the most common vaccines and vaccinations, especially for children. "It's not the vaccines that are the problem—it's the additives," says Northeastern University pharmacy professor Richard Deth. Most physicians are not even aware these additives exist, much less that they pose a problem.

Common vaccine additives include mercury, aluminum, formaldehyde, MSG, sulfites, and ethylene glycol (antifreeze). Each one of these additives has been linked to disorders ranging from brain and nerve damage to autism and attention deficit/hyperactivity disorder (ADHD). The overall amount of mercury that children typically receive from vaccinations early in life represents their entire lifetime's safe amount of mercury exposure. Symptoms of mercury toxicity in children have been documented as resembling symptoms of ADHD and autism.

"Few people realize that when they are getting a vaccine, not only are they getting a dose of the 'named' antigen or disease they're getting vaccinated against, such as diphtheria, but also a mixture of known toxic, brain-damaging, and cancer-promoting chemicals thrown in as preservatives and 'adjuvants,' which help to elicit an early, high, and long-lasting immune response," notes Paula Baillie-Hamilton, the British toxins and vaccines expert. "Ever since mass vaccinations of infants began in the twentieth century, reports of serious brain, cardiovascular, metabolic, and other injuries started filling pages of medical journals. Reports from several countries show that vaccinated children, in addition to having a lower IQ, also have a higher incidence of behavioral problems, asthma, and diabetes than unvaccinated children."

These reports of problems associated with vaccinations prompted J. Anthony Morris, former chief vaccine control officer for the FDA, to declare, "There is a great deal of evidence to prove that immunization of children does more harm than good."

At least nine childhood vaccinations are commonly required in each of the fifty states before a child can enter the public education system. These vaccine additives challenge young metabolisms and immune systems that weren't designed—not that any of ours were—to process synthetic chemicals, so the toxins are shunted off by the liver to accumulate in organs and tissues. Numerous studies in the *Journal of Applied Microbiology* and other science journals have linked one of the most common vaccine preservatives, thimerosal, to a range of toxic side effects because it contains mercury.

At a time in 1991 when public health agencies were recommending vaccinations containing thimerosal for infants, a prominent vaccinologist sent a memo warning executives at Merck, one of the drugmakers using thimerosal, that "the mercury load appears rather large" for the six-month-olds receiving the shots. Their mercury dose from thimerosal was up to eighty-seven times higher than government guidelines for the maximum daily consumption of mercury from fish.

Eight years passed before federal health officials finally decided that routine vaccinations could pose a health threat to infants. Even then the government only took the step of advising manufacturers to "consider" taking thimerosal out of vaccines. Merck did later introduce a mercury-free hepatitis B vaccine.

At a conference on vaccine safety in 2000, attended by fifty-one scientists and physicians from government and the drug industry, a Centers for Disease Control and Prevention specialist on immunizations admitted that "there is a growing recognition that cumulative exposure [to mercury in vaccines] may exceed safety guidelines." He was referring specifically to thimerosal and its effects on children, the elderly, the chronically ill, people with nutritional deficiencies, and those on certain medications.

Later in a commentary on this conference, Russell Blaylock decried how the collection of vaccine experts could only seem to agree that "as a long-term goal it was desirable to remove mercury from vaccines because it is a potentially preventable source of exposure." The words *desirable* and *long-term* were particularly offensive to Blaylock because study data had been presented that thimerosal can possibly cause several neurodevelopmental disorders, one being attention deficit disorder.

"They are all fully aware that tiny babies are receiving doses that exceed even EPA safety limits, yet all they can say is that we must 'try to remove thimerosal as soon as possible,' " fumed Blaylock. "Do they not worry about the tens of millions of babies that will continue receiving thimerosal-containing vaccines?"

The most obvious solution would be to use single-dose vials so preservatives like thimerosal would no longer be necessary. But vaccine makers resist this option because it would raise costs, which they keep down by preserving vaccines in bulk quantities. Besides, vaccine executives argue, there is "uncertainty" in the research data about the toxicity of preservatives.

"What they are admitting," continued Blaylock, "is that we have a form of mercury that has been used in vaccines since the 1930s and no one has bothered to study its effects on . . . the brain[s] of infants. Only when such problems become obvious—that is, of epidemic proportion—and the legal profession becomes involved, do they [the vaccinologists] even notice there was a problem. This is a recurring theme in the government's regulatory agencies, as witnessed with fluoride, aspartame, MSG, dioxin, and pesticides issues."

MYTHS WE CHERISH

DRUGS HAVE EXTENDED OUR LIFE SPANS

We know that people are living longer than ever before in recorded history. Most of us can see the evidence by tracing back through three or four generations of our lineage and noticing how life spans have been extended.

Pharmaceutical companies have understandably been eager to take credit for this life extension, calling their synthetic chemical creations the source of our "fountain of youth and longevity." But the real success story concerns the economic, social, and lifestyle changes that have brought about longer lives for most of us.

At the turn of the twentieth century the average life span was about forty years of age in developed countries. By the beginning of the twenty-first century life spans were nearing eighty years on average.

Of those forty years of increased life span gained during the twentieth century, no more than seven years can be credited to modern medicine, with even most of those due to advances in medical technology rather than drugs. That estimate comes from Dick Jackson, director of the National Center for Environmental Health at the Centers for Disease Control and Prevention.

"Ninety percent of the reduction in the death rate occurred before the introduction of antibiotics or vaccines," adds Anthony Cortese, a former United States Public Health Service official. "It was largely due to improved water, food, and milk sanitations; a reduction in physical crowding; the introduction of central heating, municipal sewer systems, and refrigeration; and the move away from highly toxic coal and wood burning to less-toxic natural gas and oil."

The scientist who discovered the first two commercially manufactured antibiotics, the microbiologist Rene Dubos, admitted in his book *The Mirage of Health*: "The introduction of inexpensive cotton undergarments easy to launder and of transparent glass that brought light into the most humble dwelling contributed more to the control of infection than did all the drugs and medical practices."

Modern medical technology certainly plays an important role in extending lives, with heart bypass surgery, pacemakers, life-support systems for the lungs, kidney dialysis machines, and the whole range of other marvels. By contrast, synthetic chemical drugs play, at best, a supporting role in this process.

We can only begin to imagine how much longer our average life spans might become if our immune systems were to remain strong and vigorous, our diets free of toxins and full of nutrients, and our minds and bodies no longer under constant assault by synthetic chemical invaders.

DISTURBING TREND NUMBER ONE

OVERMEDICATING OUR CHILDREN

Because children have lower body weights and less-developed metabolisms, they are more vulnerable to toxic effects from synthetic chemicals. That makes this news from Texas all the more disturbing: Children as young as three years old are being forced to take mind-altering drugs by Child Protective Service employees in that state. An investigation by a San Antonio television station in 2004 discovered that two out of every three foster children in Texas had been placed on psychotropic medications, many of them on two or more such drugs. One child was being forced to take seventeen different prescription drugs to alter or regulate behavior and sleep. At least three hundred children under the age of seven were found to be on multiple mood and behavior medications.

After the FDA approved a medication called Ritalin in 1961 for use by children diagnosed with behavior problems, more than one hundred thousand kids were taking the drug within a decade. By the mid 1980s, one million children were on Ritalin. By the turn of the century, *six million* children in the United States were Ritalin users. Of that number, nearly half were also being medicated for attention deficit/hyperactivity disorder (ADHD).

A 2005 study by the Centers for Disease Control and Prevention raised the alarm that for the first time, as many children in the United States are now being treated for ADHD as are being medicated for asthma. Among males twelve years of age nearly 10 percent have been diagnosed with ADHD, which is defined as a neurobehavioral disorder characterized by the inability to pay attention, accompanied by hyperactivity and impulsivity. "This is a disorder that is really taking a very substantial toll on society," observed David Marks, a psychologist with the ADHD Center at Mount Sinai Medical Center in New York. "In adulthood individuals with ADHD miss more work, they're more likely to get fired, they're more likely to receive negative work reviews. It does constitute a very substantial health burden."

What is happening to an entire generation of our children? For one thing, there is evidence that Ritalin use in the long term may actually be exacerbating a condition caused by other synthetic chemicals. A study published in *The Journal of Biological Psychiatry* found that high doses of vitamin B_6 did a better job of reducing hyperactivity in children than Ritalin and at a far lower cost and with far fewer side effects. Yet, physicians continue prescribing the drug to ever greater numbers of kids by telling parents "your child is abnormal and this drug is a replacement therapy," as though the drug itself were a naturally occurring chemical in the brain.

DISTURBING TREND NUMBER TWO
THE MARKETING OF DISEASE

It was a surgeon, Susan Love, who first exposed a drug industry secret when she was widely quoted as saying, "Marketing a disease is the best way to market a drug."

Osteoporosis, a thinning of the bones, became one of the first diseases thrust upon the U.S. public as part of a marketing scheme. As described by John Abramson, the drug manufacturer Wyeth-Ayerst hired a public relations firm to stimulate public concern in 1985 about osteoporosis so the company could offer its estrogen therapy drug, Premarin, as an antidote. Sales of Premarin had been lagging before this campaign began, but the public relations effect of stirring up fears increased sales of the drug by 40 percent the first year.

Since then drug advertising has been designed to evoke emotional responses in viewers and readers. We are seeing this trend in the marketing of drugs for type 2 diabetes, for attention deficit disorder, and for erectile dysfunction. Even more recent is the "female sexual dysfunction" campaign promoting the hormone testosterone and Viagra for women, which prompted a rebuke of Pfizer and other drug companies by the *British Medical Journal* for "a corporate-sponsored creation of a disease."

Given that only a small percentage of new pharmaceutical drug brands introduced into the marketplace each year actually contain new ingredients, it should not surprise us that the drug industry keeps the pressure on itself to create disease industries to revitalize its older or lower-selling drugs. But once we begin to appreciate the impact this marketing strategy is having on our pocketbooks and on our health, we learn how truly pernicious a grip Big Pharma has on us. That theme came across impressively in the book *Generation Rx: How Prescription Drugs Are Altering American Lives, Minds, and Bodies,* by Greg Critser, whose previous book was *Fat Land.*

Big Pharma has been targeting specific age groups, called "pharmaceutical tribes," to advance their disease-racket marketing plans. Some examples are "The Tribe of High Performance Youth" who ingest prescription drug concoctions nicknamed "California Cocktails" consisting of Ritalin, Neurontin, and Wellbutrin, treatments respectively for attention deficit, epilepsy, and depression. Or the "Tribe of High Performance Aging," those middle-aged pill poppers trying to extend their life spans.

A result is that half of all Americans take at least one prescription drug every day. Many of them consume three or more every day. No wonder we are experiencing an epidemic of liver disease. We are overwhelming our livers, kidneys, and stomachs with prescription drug combinations that produce synergies no one has ever calculated or studied.

In his book, Critser quotes an expert on child psychopharmacology, Glen Elliott, who despairs at what Big Pharma is doing to an entire generation of youth: "The problem is that our usage has outstripped our knowledge base. Let's face it, we're experimenting on these kids without tracking the results."

DISTURBING TREND NUMBER THREE
WE NO LONGER KNOW WHAT TO EXPECT

Bizarre case: A medicine called ivermectin, given to cows, sheep, and horses as protection from parasites, has turned their dung into a toxic and virtually indestructible health hazard in the French Alps. Insects die once in contact with the toxic dung, and birds and bats eat the insects and then sicken and die. "We have seen cowpats [cow dung] survive four years or more," marveled Jean-Pierre Lumaret of the University of Montpellier. "If the dung does not decompose, it becomes like stone, which stops the grass from growing."

More bizarre case: A drug called Mirapex, approved by the FDA in

1997, to relieve tremors and stiffness in Parkinson's patients, has been found to cause compulsive behaviors as a side effect. *Archives of Neurology* reported in July 2005 that some Mirapex users became compulsive gamblers and lost large sums of money in casinos and playing the lottery. Other users developed compulsive sex addictions that destroyed their marriages, or they became compulsive shoppers and went heavily into debt.

Even more bizarre: New regulatory rules on human testing to determine health risks from pesticides and other drug exposures were adopted in September 2005 by the EPA to allow experimentation on "abused and neglected children" without the permission of parents or guardians. Absolutely anyone can be subjected to "ethically deficient" research, so the regulatory language reads, if the EPA determines it to be "crucial to protect public health." There was surprisingly little public attention or outcry when these rules were announced.

As a result of a century of innovations in synthetic chemical manufacturing, we have inherited a virtually indestructible residue of toxins in the environment. Synthetic chemicals have seared into nature a seemingly immortal stamp. Whether they are pesticides or pharmaceutical drugs, what all of these synthetic chemicals set loose among us have in common is the identity of having been conceived by chemists and birthed in laboratories to be "magic bullets." They were intended to either kill something, preserve something, clean something, or mask the symptoms of something. Now we must consider the prospect that some of these chemicals will survive longer than the species who created them.

CHAPTER SIX

ARE WE BECOMING A MUTANT SPECIES?

"Exposure to toxic chemicals and a combination of genetic and toxic chemical factors cause about 28 percent of all developmental defects affecting 120,000 infants born each year."

—National Research Council Commission
on Life Sciences study, 2000

In the moments following the birth of Sue Green's first baby everything seemed normal, but then the mood suddenly shifted. "The midwife was smiling, then her face fell," remembers Sue. " 'Congratulations,' she said. 'It's a . . . ' And then there was silence."

Over the next few hours this awkward silence continued as a parade of doctors and nurses came to view the child. Finally, overcome with anxiety, Sue demanded an explanation. "You're not telling me something!" she screamed. "Is it a boy or a girl?" No one could tell her.

So began a heartbreaking article in *The Times* of London (July 26, 2005) by Steve Boggan that described how a couple in Northern Ireland, Sue and John Green, spent four weeks consulting with specialists and putting their baby through chromosome tests in an effort to establish whether the child was a boy or a girl.

Rather than just aberrations, these sorts of reproductive disorders have become a horrifyingly routine chapter in the annals of modern medicine, according to *The Times*, leading some prominent scientists to blame endocrine disrupters, a class of synthetic chemicals that show up everywhere in our plastics, fabrics, carpets, perfumes, pesticides sprayed on food crops, and a host of other products. Laboratory tests have shown they can disrupt the delicate balance of hormones in the human body, especially when exposure occurs in the fetus. The wide range of effects on reproductive health and gender identity is only now being documented and measured.

A group of 120 scientists from around the world met in Prague in May 2005 and issued a warning and an appeal to all governments to acknowledge their "serious concern about the high prevalence of reproductive disorders in European boys and young men." These health specialists identified endocrine-disrupter chemicals as the prime suspect for the epidemic of reproductive abnormalities being seen worldwide.

Studies in *Pediatrics* and other medical journals reveal that since the early 1960s there has been an estimated 40 percent increase in male infants born in Europe and the United States with abnormal penises and symptoms of feminization. Other health statistics tell a similar reproductive horror story.

- At least 10 percent of all couples in the United States are unable to conceive a child, and the numbers seem to be growing. Some communities in Canada report precipitous declines in male births, down to just one-third of all births. In the last two decades of the twentieth century, a 400 percent increase in tubal pregnancies was reported among women in developed nations.
- In vitro fertilization clinics throughout the United States report a huge spike in the number of abnormal embryos being produced by young, healthy women in their twenties who should be in the prime of their reproductive lives. Nearly 80 percent of three hundred embryos sampled were abnormal, according to the authors of a study on reproduction who presented their alarming results to an October 2005 conference in Montreal of the American Society for Reproductive Medicine and the Canadian Fertility and Andrology Society. The genetic defect rate among fertile women could prove to be far higher, because only eleven chromosomes were tested for this study. Experts specu-

lated that "environmental factors"—a euphemism for synthetic chemicals—might be causing the rapid and widespread degeneration.

- Male sperm counts worldwide have been reduced by 50 percent in the past half century, and during the same period testicular cancer rates underwent a 600 percent increase. In China, the fastest-developing country in the world, a 2001 study found that 85 percent of university students tested were infertile.

The list of statistics demonstrating an unmistakable pattern that something is going seriously wrong goes on and on. Some of these developments might at first seem rather humorous if the implications weren't so grim.

During the summer of 2005 clinics in London began reporting an upsurge in the numbers of men seeking breast reduction surgery. In just a year clinics throughout the city had more than doubled their male clientele for breast reduction treatment. "Hormones contained in the food we eat may be one of the reasons for the increase," speculated Yannis Alexandrides, a London surgeon who told *The Sunday Times* that he now performs one male breast reduction surgery a week, compared to one a month just a few years earlier. Other physicians told the newspaper they suspected that female hormones from contraceptive pills, flushed through sewage systems and recycled into tap water, could be the culprit in demasculinizing so many grown men.

Among eight-year-old girls in the United States, Britain, and Australia, one out of every six has already entered puberty, with breast growth, pubic hair, and even menstruation. Just a generation ago only one out of every one hundred eight-year-old girls had entered puberty, whereas today nearly two out of every one hundred girls are showing sexual development *at three years of age*! This phenomenon has come to be known as "precocious puberty." A study in the journal *Nature* determined that the onset of puberty before age ten more than doubles a female's chances of breast cancer and ovarian cancer later in life.

What is equally astounding to me are the elaborate rationalizations embraced by many Western physicians and the medical establishment to explain these extraordinarily rapid changes in sexual development. They claim that precocious puberty is nothing more than a natural by-product of improved nutrition. They try to reassure parents that their daughters' experience of "raging hormones" and menstruation at age eight shouldn't be a cause for concern because it is now considered normal for puberty to ·begin at that age. What they are confessing is that synthetic chemicals are redefining what it means to be normal.

To try to understand what is going on, let's start with the word *hormone*, which comes from Greek and means "to set in motion." That is what hormones do, they activate our metabolic processes. Our hormones in turn are regulated by the endocrine system, a series of glands that include the pituitary, pineal, thyroid, adrenal, hypothalamus, parathyroid, pancreas, ovaries, and testes.

Endocrine system disrupter chemicals imitate our natural hormones by affecting any or all of the glands that produce the hormones. This can trigger or disrupt our natural hormone production. Estrogens associated with the reproductive system are especially vulnerable to disrupter chemicals, sometimes called "gender-bender" synthetics. More than fifty chemicals in common usage, ranging from plasticizers to pesticides, have been identified as hormone disrupters. Dozens more are candidates.

A report on endocrine disrupters (also called hormonally active agents or HAAs) prepared by the National Research Council, an arm of the National Academy of Sciences, did authoritatively conclude in 1999 that "adverse reproductive and developmental effects have been observed in human populations, wildlife, and laboratory animals as a consequence of exposure to HAAs."

PCBs, DDT, dioxin, and dozens more synthetic toxins are stored in the fatty tissues of fish and other animals and then passed on to the humans who consume them. "These persistent chemicals fake their way into the endocrine system, masquerading as hormones," write the three authors of the book *Affluenza*. "It's a deadly case of miscommunication. When hormones, our chemical messengers, are released or suppressed at the wrong time in the wrong amounts, life gets bent out of shape."

CANARIES IN A COAL MINE

If we treat fish and other animals in the wild as comparable to canaries in a coal mine, able to alert us by their distress to invisible dangers, we find ourselves surrounded by an accumulation of evidence for something having gone seriously wrong in nature. We have been given a fair and prolonged warning. Those patterns of abnormalities we now see in our human species started appearing with increasing frequency among species of wildlife several decades ago.

Hermaphrodite fish began turning up in the Great Lakes (also turning many of the offspring of the seagulls that ate them into hermaphrodites) about the same time as feminized wildlife made an appearance in Florida's Lake Apopka, where male alligators have been born without phalluses and turtles have hatched with intersex (both male and female) sex organs. Hermaphrodite shellfish have been turning up along the northeastern coast of Chesapeake Bay. A high proportion of wild chinook salmon in the Columbia River of Washington state have reversed their sex, switching their sexual characteristics from male to female. In 84 percent of fish tested, chromosomal males had female reproductive tracts. Concentrations of estrogen-mimic chemicals such as plasticizers and the pesticide atrazine were detected in the river.

Along the Potomac River in Maryland at least 60 percent of fish examined by scientists in 2003 and 2004 had mutated into hermaphrodites or from male to female, with the fish born male having eggs growing inside their testes. Numerous pharmaceutical drugs that had passed unaltered through sewage treatment plants were detected in the river. "We might just be seeing the tip of the iceberg in terms of the cumulative impact of all this," commented Thomas Burke, associate chairman of health policy at the Johns Hopkins Bloomberg School of Public Health in Baltimore. These findings were particularly alarming because Washington, D.C., and other cities along the Potomac draw their drinking water from the river.

Similar mutations have been showing up across the United States. In testing done by Baylor University biologists monitoring a Denton, Texas, creek, male minnows were found to have mutated in the presence of birth control medications discharged by a wastewater plant. As the nation's use of Prozac doubled since 2000, to be consumed by fifty-four million people, more than half of all streams and rivers tested by the United States Geological Survey show residues of this antidepressant drug, which is affecting growth and reproduction in clams, mussels, and fish. At the University of Georgia, environmental health professor Marsha Black discovered that Prozac affects fish in Georgia and Mississippi rivers at extremely low concentrations, less than one part per billion, which is about like an aspirin in a tank of one million gallons of water. Nearly half of drug-exposed fish were dying prematurely, others were growth-stunted or mutated, and still more swam around in circles endlessly in disoriented confusion.

Off the coast of Southern California sewage effluent has been deforming the sex organs of marine life. About one billion gallons of wastewater is discharged every day through undersea pipelines into deep waters off Los Angeles and Orange counties. During 2005 the Southern California Coastal Water Research Project caught and analyzed hundreds of bottom-dwelling fish from that area and found two-thirds of some species had become intersex fish, with both male and female reproductive organs. The ocean floor's sediment was found to be contaminated with estrogenic chemicals that bottom-feeding organisms absorb and pass along up the food chain.

The entire male fish population of many European rivers has been feminized as well. "We are finding this problem right across northern Europe; it is clearly widespread," says Alan Pickering of Britain's Natural Environment Research Council. Freshwater fish in five out of seven northern European countries showed reproductive abnormalities from exposure to endocrine-disrupting chemicals present in sewage effluents. In the River Aire in Yorkshire, 100 percent of the male fish have been feminized by gender-bender chemicals.

We might try to shrug off these accounts by labeling them aberrations or perverse material for science fiction. But even a casual reading of the scientific documentation of this trend makes for a sober awakening. One of the first authoritative alerts came in 1993, when a science paper published in *The Lancet* revealed a pattern of fish and alligators in the wild being demasculinized from contact with bodies of water containing the female hormone estrogen.

The herbicide atrazine, used to control weeds, has been found to be the cause of demasculinized frogs even at extraordinarily low levels of exposure. A 2002 report in *Proceedings of the National Academy of Sciences* discovered that at exposure levels far lower than those normally found in lakes, rivers, streams, and drinking water, frogs had their hormones disrupted by molecules of atrazine. Levels as low as 0.1 parts per billion caused frogs to become hermaphrodites. Under EPA regulations, atrazine levels of three parts per billion are allowed in drinking water.

A study in *Nature* (2002) produced evidence that amphibians in the wild are being "chemically castrated," as biologist Tyrone Hayes put it. In areas where atrazine had been applied, 100 percent of male frogs were found with abnormal sex organs. The findings in this study were later replicated by four other research teams.

Low doses of a fungicide called vindozolin, at levels of just a few parts per million, have been found to profoundly alter sexual development in male rats, reducing sperm counts by 90 percent and producing feminization and other deformities. "There is every reason to conclude that the effect translates over into humans," wrote the four authors of a 1999 study in the journal *Toxicology & Industrial Health*.

The chemical and pesticide industries have ridiculed these and other related scientific studies. A common attack has been to claim that plants also naturally produce estrogen-mimic chemicals and this could account for reported birth anomalies, though no explanation has been offered as to why plants might have suddenly started trying to poison us.

That industry explanation drew a response from the team of scientists who authored the book *Our Stolen Future* and who continue to maintain a Web site devoted to endocrine-disrupter chemicals. They point out that synthetic hormone mimics pose an even greater hazard than natural compounds "because they can persist in the body for years, while plant estrogens might be eliminated within a day."

We should also place this epidemic of reproductive abnormalities in the context of the broader patterns being observed worldwide. The American Museum of Natural History conducted a nationwide survey of biologists and found seven out of every ten believe "we are in the midst of a mass extinction of living things and this dramatic loss of species poses a major threat to human existence. . . . This mass extinction is the fastest in

Earth's 4.5-billion-year history and, unlike prior extinctions, is mainly the result of human activity."

PLASTICS ARE HARMLESS

An area of the central Pacific Ocean about the size of Africa—around ten million square miles—has become a virtual museum for the debris of our civilization's synthetics paradigm. In this region circular winds produce circular ocean currents, and as a result, anything that floats and has washed down rivers into the sea ends up collecting here in the planet's largest garbage dump. Oceanographers who have visited and studied the region have discovered that this huge section of water, down to a depth of thirty meters, is choked with plastics.

Everything from cheap plastic fishing nets to plastic cups and plastic cigarette lighters can be found floating in congealing heaps. Unlike the flotsam of civilization that typically collected here a half century ago, this plastic waste doesn't biodegrade and eventually disappear into the environment. Instead, plastic goes through a process called *photo-degrading*, in which sunlight breaks it down into smaller pieces until it becomes individual molecules of plastic polymers.

"Plastic, like diamonds, are forever!" quips Charles Moore, captain of the oceanographic research vessel *Alguita*, operated by the Algalita Marine Research Foundation in Long Beach, California. "My research has documented six pounds of plastic for every pound of plankton in this area."

Mile-long streams of this debris periodically drift to the Hawaiian Islands and coat the beaches in shreds of blue-green plastic. Aquatic life such as sea turtles and many species of fish commonly mistake the stuff for their natural food. Underwater photographers have captured images of transparent aquatic organisms with colorful plastic fragments visible in their bellies. In the October 2005 issue of *National Geographic* an albatross chick was pictured on an island beach after having died at age six months from starvation due to a full stomach. It had consumed hundreds of plastic pieces—from cigarette lighters to clothespins—until its stomach was full and it couldn't ingest any nutrients.

What makes this situation even more perilous is what plastic polymers attract. "As these fragments float around," says Moore, "they accumulate the poisons we manufacture that are not water soluble. It turns out that plastic polymers are sponges for DDT, PCBs, and nonylphenols—oily toxics that don't dissolve in seawater. Plastic pellets have been found to accumulate up to one million times the level of these poisons that are floating in the water itself. . . . Hormone receptors cannot distinguish these toxics from the natural estrogenic hormone, estradiol . . . our worst pollutants are being ingested by the most efficient natural vacuum cleaners nature ever invented. . . . These organisms are in turn eaten by fish and then, in many cases, by humans. The whole issue of hormone disruption is becoming one of, if not the biggest, environmental issues of the twenty-first century."

Between 1965 and 1995 the amount of plastic produced in the world went from two million tons a year to more than twenty-four million tons. By 2000 we were producing about one hundred million tons. In the United States alone, production increased almost 10 percent from just 2003 to 2004. It promises to escalate in quantum leaps as "new plastics are in the works with even more impossible qualities," according to *U.S. News & World Report*.

Using the building blocks of matter, such as hydrogen, nitrogen, and carbon, plastics are formed with the addition of chemical catalysts, massive pressure, and intense heat or cold. Mega molecules called polymers emerge, and these are then molded into desired shapes. They are virtually indestructible, and the new plastics being introduced into products will even have the ability to "heal" themselves because if they are cracked open by age or wear, microcapsules inside the material itself will release fresh supplies of polymers to reconstitute itself.

"It is the Rasputin of modern materials," marvels Stephen Fenichell, author of *Plastic: The Making of a Synthetic Century*. "You can break it, chop it, dice it, shred it, burn it, and bury it, but it stubbornly refuses to die."

Some types of plastic molecules enter the human body and also stubbornly refuse to die. Bisphenol A (BPA) is used to manufacture the polycarbonate plastics added to food containers, baby bottles, and a range of other products. Blood and urine sampling by the Centers for Disease

Control and Prevention discovered BPA in 95 percent of all people in the United States, apparently the result of BPA leaching from food products. "Toxicologic studies of laboratory animals suggest that exposure to BPA is associated with reproductive anomalies," says a report by the National Center for Environmental Health, a branch of the Centers for Disease Control and Prevention.

A laboratory accident in 1998 unexpectedly revealed the extent to which BPA might impact health. At Case Western Reserve University in Cleveland, a lab assistant mistakenly cleaned the cages of laboratory animals with a detergent commonly used on floors. Plastic in the cages reacted to the detergent and leached BPA into the animals' food and water. Nearly half of the offspring born to the affected animals had chromosomal abnormalities. As one might hope under the circumstances, at this point some scientists became concerned about the possible effects of BPA on human health since it is a chemical found in products that keep our food fresh, our floors shiny, our fabrics stain-free, and has a myriad of other uses that make life more convenient.

Subsequent studies of BPA have shown it to alter fetal mouse development and cause reproductive abnormalities at an extraordinarily low dosage, just two parts per billion. That is the molecular equivalent of two credit cards lying in the middle of an area the size of several hundred football fields.

Plastic linings are found in about 85 percent of the food cans sold in the United States. Several scientists from the University of Granada in Spain analyzed twenty brands of this canned food and found BPA contamination in half of all they examined. Some BPA in cans of corn and other food was found to be in amounts of eighty parts per billion, far in excess of the level a Stanford University research team had previously identified as causing breast cancer cells to proliferate.

A group of professors at the Yale School of Medicine reported in 2005 that low doses of BPA, as found in food-storage containers, textiles, and flame retardants, may lead to learning disabilities and age-related neurodegenerative diseases in humans. While their study, published in the journal *Environmental Health Perspectives*, used low doses of BPA in female rats, they claim the observed effects in areas of the brain involved with the formation and retention of memory can be extrapolated to humans. They speculate that BPAs may be a causative factor in the development of Alzheimer's disease, now afflicting nearly five million Americans, and in learning disabilities in children. When corrected for body size differences, the BPA effects seen in lab animals are within the range of what we humans normally ingest or inhale from the leaching that occurs in our use of plastics in everyday products.

Plastics also contribute to gender-bender characteristics. Medical researchers at the University of Rochester in New York, writing in a 2005 issue of *Environmental Health Perspectives*, explained how an examination of 134 boys found sex abnormalities, ranging from small testicles to abnormally small penises, in those whose mothers had higher-than-normal levels of phthalate-related chemicals in their blood. It didn't take large exposures to these chemicals for them to produce the observed effects.

Phthalates (pronounced "thallets") appear in everything from children's plastic toys to drugs, cosmetics, and insecticides. They are made from petroleum by-products and turn rigid plastics into pliable plastics. Worldwide, industries use five million metric tons of phthalates each year, so it's no wonder these molecules show up in human body fluids and tissues. Industry trade association groups such as the American Chemistry Council claim that after a half century of use phthalates have never been proven to cause any health problems for a single human being.

That's a huge claim to make and, if true, would make phthalates practically unique among all synthetic-chemical creations. But chinks are beginning to appear in this armor of perceived safety and respectability. A 2003 study, for example, conducted by researchers at the Harvard School of Public Health, examined 168 male patients at a fertility clinic, measuring phthalate levels in their urine. Those men with the highest levels turned out to be up to five times more likely to have low sperm counts or low sperm activity essential to fertilization. A second study raising concerns about phthalates and reproductive health appeared in 2005, authored by scientists at the University of Copenhagen. They examined ninety-six baby boys and found the ones with abnormally low testosterone had been fed breast milk containing high levels of phthalates their mothers had absorbed from everyday plastic products.

These studies raised enough alarms that Japan banned certain phthalates from food-handling equipment in schools, and the European Union banned some types of phthalates from toys and cosmetics. By contrast, U.S. phthalate use continues to grow as the plastics and chemical industries loudly insist that we have nothing to worry about, that everything is normal.

Their dismissive attitude and posturing is perfectly understandable—though hardly defensible—because these industries are so dependent on the chemicals that medical science is calling into question. Corporate profits are at stake, and to even admit a health concern about their products would open them up to liability lawsuits. They are mostly stuck in a position of stubborn resistance to any scientific evidence that undermines the public's faith in the benefits and safety of the synthetics belief system.

MYTHS WE CHERISH
EVERYTHING IS NORMAL

More people seem to have cancer today only because we are living longer. More children seem to have autism today only because our detection techniques for disease are more highly developed. More of us may have more chemicals detectable in our bodies today, but that is normal and not a cause for concern because those chemicals are "just passing through."

Those three statements—each of which is countered somewhere in this book—are a sampling of informational "facts" featured on Web sites funded by the chemical industry and the plastics manufacturers. They typify the well-funded public relations campaign initiated by those economic interests, along with the food and drug industries, to convince us that we have nothing to fear but fear itself.

The "just passing through" analogy in particular, as promoted on the Phthalates Information Center site, is intriguing enough to quote at length. "According to movies about the Old West, the town sheriff made it a habit to ask strangers in town about their intentions. The response 'just passing through' was meant to reassure the sheriff and the local populace the stranger wanted no trouble and would soon be gone. 'Just passing through' could be the exit line for most of the substances that get into our bodies from our daily eating, drinking, breathing, and touching."

Chemicals that we carry around within us as a body burden, according to this plastics industry argument, are well below regulatory safety levels and break down and disappear as fast as they arrive. "Just like the cinematic sheriff, the body can readily handle the small amounts of materials that are just passing through." In other words, don't worry, be happy. Those seven hundred or so synthetic chemicals a normal person now carries around in their body (which hadn't, by the way, broken down and disappeared when they were measured in the Centers for Disease Control and Prevention studies) have become normal hitchhikers in our bodies today, even though none of these chemicals even existed when your grandparents were born.

Redefining what is normal has become a game that special interests play. But the rules of this game are changing faster than anyone wants to acknowledge. Take the most basic assumption in chemical-risk assessment—an assumption used in connection with all products produced—that there is a certain safe level of contamination below which no effects are caused. That reassuring idea was dealt a serious blow in 1999 with the publication, in *Environmental Health Perspectives*, of a study showing that endocrine disrupter chemicals can cause health effects at extremely low dosages. Some low levels of exposure actually create more negative health effects in either humans or animals than higher doses do.

A friend of mine, Terry Cafferty, a senior engineering consultant to various aerospace firms, heard some of these "redefining what is normal" statements from the chemical industry and detected some parallels to his own field. "I often deal with scientists in my work, really intelligent people who are designing and conducting very elaborate experiments to try to find out how everything came to be. They are, underneath their highly specialized education and training, very ordinary people with families and ordinary lives. They are not infallible sources of truth and wisdom. They disagree with each other."

"There is an erroneous and widespread perception about scientists, namely that they are completely wise and can therefore be relied upon to tell 'the truth.' They are supposed to be 'objective' observers of 'objective' reality. Scientists and doctors are subjective beings like everyone else, and their opinions, feelings, and perceptions 'color' how they see the objective facts of any question or situation.

"Given that the science of low-level chemical exposure is in its infancy (and the science of low-level synergy is barely conceived), is it more reasonable to take the side of caution? Is it more reasonable to imagine that the human immune system doesn't know what to do with synthetics, and so they are stored in the body, leading to increasing toxicity and disease? Or is it reasonable to assume you can put low levels of anything in there, as long as it has not been proven to cause a problem?

"Scientists do not say that low levels of chemicals in the human body are harmless. What they say is that many of them have not been proven harmless or harmful by means that satisfy them. Does that mean they are personally anxious to ingest a bunch of different chemicals into their bodies because it has not been proven harmful to do so? I doubt it. But the mind game they continue to play with the public goes like this: 'It hasn't been proven that ingesting (or inhaling or absorbing) low levels of a synthetic chemical is harmful to your health. So therefore you should go ahead and keep on ingesting and absorbing this stuff until science gets around to convincingly proving that it is OK.' This is dangerous nonsense. These guys are saying trace levels of chemical X may not be causative in relation to an increase in disease. But what about trace levels of ten, twenty, fifty, or one hundred chemicals? What are the synergistic effects that cause illness and disease? Do these scientists know? Of course not! But any idiot knows that if you pollute yourself, you get sick."

Responding to skeptics who discount as alarmist all concerns about the hormonal effects of synthetic chemicals, the authors of *Our Stolen Future* point out that "manufacturers frequently withhold information about the ingredients in their products using the claim of proprietary information or trade secrets." As a result, "it is anybody's guess how many of the plastic consumer goods on the market contain hormone-disrupting chemicals. The information in the scientific literature about the biological activity of and human exposure to chemicals of concern is equally fragmentary and unsatisfactory."

What is definitely *not* normal is how our bodies are losing many of our natural defenses that help to repel chemical and viral invaders, and to keep us healthy. A 2004 special issue of *Environmental Science & Technology*, an American Chemical Society journal, was devoted to the new science of ecotoxicology, the study of synthetic-chemical effects on life and the environment. The journal editors wrote that this new field and its research are vital "if we are to protect our living heritage from the cocktail of chemicals present in all environments." Cited as particularly important was research about the impact of musk fragrances, those synthetic chemicals used to enhance the smell of shampoos and air fresheners and detergents, which aren't removed by sewage treatment and as a result now contaminate most bodies of water.

A California Sea Grant program examined how these synthetic fragrances affect the natural defenses of mussels. After a large group of mussels was exposed to low concentrations of six commercial musk chemicals, they were washed and placed in water containing a red dye. The mussels quickly soaked up the dye, which was abnormal because mussels have the ability to detect and repel foreign substances, such as dyes. They had lost their natural defense as a result of the musk chemical exposure.

Like mussels and most other animal species, humans use protective mechanisms against chemical invaders. It is known that these musk chemicals are building up in human tissues and becoming a permanent part of our toxic body burden. The health dangers are unknown, just another unknown among many, but this study suggests a way in which these chemicals may be weakening the human immune system. This is definitely not normal.

MYTHS WE CHERISH

ANIMAL TESTING PREDICTS HUMAN HEALTH

Let's ponder the implications of a big monkey wrench that has been thrown into the idea that we can consistently predict much of anything about dangers to human health based on animal experimentation results.

Two books by anesthesiologist C. Ray Greek and veterinarian Jean Swingle Greek, *Specious Science* (2003) and *Sacred Cows and Golden Geese* (2000), present devastating evidence that animal studies not only fail to accurately predict how drugs or toxins will affect humans, but that experimental results from animals often mislead scientists and harm human patients.

Here are a few of the many dozens of examples the authors cite:

- The popular diet drug fen-phen passed all its animal tests for safety, but once humans began using it the discovery was made (as a result of death and illness) that it damaged the human heart but not animal hearts. The arthritis drug Opren passed all of its tests on monkeys, but then it killed sixty-one humans before it was withdrawn from the market. A drug called Cylert worked well in rats for symptoms of attention deficit/hyperactivity disorder but when given to children caused liver failure in thirteen of them before it was withdrawn.
- Tobacco companies claimed that cigarette smoking was safe because in their lab studies rats didn't contract lung cancer, but several decades of epidemiological study of humans has determined that people's lungs are susceptible to cigarette smoke even when rat's lungs are unaffected.
- National Cancer Institute studies show that 63 percent of the time, drugs that were effective against human cancers failed to work against the same cancers in mice.
- Researchers gave animals six drugs known to have eighty-eight side effects in humans; twenty-two of these side effects also appeared in the lab animals, but other side effects common to humans failed to appear in the animals. About 76 percent of the time, the animal results had no application to human experience.

Most revealing of all has been what common household aspirin does to animals. "Our most popular drug, grandfathered in before the requirement for animal validation was legislated, would never have made it through the animal assays now required. Aspirin produces birth defects in mice, rats, guinea pigs, rabbits, cats, primates, and dogs." Nor would penicillin have made it through clinical trials for use on humans—penicillin kills guinea pigs and cats, and causes deformities in rats and many other types of test animals.

Animals are generally not good predictors of what effects chemicals will have on humans because of differences in their anatomy and physiology at the celluar level, and a range of differences in metabolism and the absorption of substances. Difficulty in dosage control and an inability of laboratory conditions to imitate normal human habits also contribute to this failure of accurate extrapolation from animal to human.

Even among humans, chemical effects differ according to genetic and environmental factors that usually cannot be predicted. The Environmental Working Group describes these variables this way: "Many factors determine how a drug, allergen, or toxic substance will affect a person—genetics, metabolism, age, sex, size, disease, diet, and environment. The result is vast variability in the human response to chemicals, viruses, drugs, and a host of substances (up to one hundred thousandfold differences), most of which is influenced by factors that individuals cannot control."

So why are animal tests still performed—and given respect—when they can be so fatally flawed? The two physicians Greek and Greek say it is because industries, the pharmaceutical companies in particular, only want "to get the substance onto the pharmacy shelves and to protect themselves legally if a problem arises." That is why experimental studies are often shortened before tests can turn up evidence of toxicity and why some researchers involved in clinical trials have been accused of underreporting drug safety problems.

Now that we know animal studies may incorrectly imply the absence of risk in humans and that animal tests showing harm may not indicate a real danger to people, where does that leave us regarding health concerns from chemical exposure? The simple answer is that we should use the results of animal tests in biomedical research as suggestive of harm or of safety and not as predictive.

This standard will obviously cut many different ways into the debate over chemical toxins and health, and it may dilute the impact of many of the experimental findings discussed on the pages of this book. But the most signficiant repercussion is the doubt this casts on the contentions of the chemical, food, drug, and other industries' testing procedures. The truth is—we simply don't know what is safe. It only makes sense to be cautious.

We now face an enormous uncertainty principle. Will what we don't know hurt us? The key to our survival will come from common sense and observation. If animals in the wild are exhibiting a general class of symptoms indicating illness and disease, and the cause and effect is confirmed by laboratory tests of other animals, and then we also see in the human population the same general but widespread class of symptoms, we can logically deduce that we have found something to be concerned about.

That is exactly the pattern we see today regarding our reproductive health. Animals in nature are experiencing reproductive abnormalities. These abnormalities have been replicated in the laboratory using the suspected chemical causation agents. Humans are experiencing many of the same symptoms observed in nature and in the laboratory. The suspected chemical causes are present everywhere around us. What additional evidence does a reasonable person need to accept the possibility that we are doing all of this to ourselves?

EVOLUTION OR EXTINCTION?

Will our future as a species be shaped more by pressures for evolution or for extinction? A team of biologists at Washington State University reported in the journal *Science* their experimental evidence that chemical toxin damage from endocrine disrupters can be inherited, passing from one generation to another as a DNA modification. Such a process could turn out to be irreversible and threaten the long-term survival of any species.

This 2005 study shook the foundations of reproductive biology because the findings suggested another route for chemical toxins to trigger the onset of disease. Though this study was performed on rats, using a common insecticide normally sprayed on cropland and a fungicide used on vineyards (both suspected endocrine disrupters), it still may apply to humans if only because the principle demonstrated was so contrary to prevailing scientific opinion. Female rats were exposed in mid-gestation to the two chemicals, and 90 percent of their male offspring were born with low sperm counts and abnormal sperm production, while the other 10 percent were completely infertile. These patterns of male infertility were then passed down to the second-, third-, and fourth-generation males, none of whom were directly exposed to the toxins. It wasn't a change in their DNA code but a change in the way their genes worked.

"That [the changes are] carried down through the generations is what's new and novel here," Paul Turek, a male-infertility specialist at the

University of California at San Francisco, told *USA Today*. "Everyone agrees that exposure of the fetus at a certain critical time can cause malformed organs and birth defects. But no one ever imagined this might persist at some level for three more generations."

Equally disturbing, males descended from females exposed to the toxins were more susceptible to other diseases, especially prostate and kidney cancer. The implications for humankind fit the patterns we are seeing with infertility and disease. "You may develop a disease state even though you never had direct exposure," concluded the study authors, "and you may pass it on to your great grandchildren. This is an epigenetic transgenerational phenomenon that impacts: (1) the potential hazards of environmental toxins, (2) provides a new variable for consideration in the development of disease, and (3) is a new factor to consider in evolutionary biology as it pertains to environmental influence on adaptive mutations and natural selection."

Mainstream medical science had previously believed that for any disease or disorder to be inherited, a gene must mutate and then be passed along to offspring. Now it has been shown that inherited reproductive disorders can be passed on from a simple chemical modification of the DNA.

Like many discoveries in science this one came about by accident. During a separate experiment, a researcher in Michael Skinner's lab inadvertently allowed two rats exposed to the pesticide and fungicide to breed. The low sperm counts and other disorders were then observed in successive generations.

"This wasn't supposed to happen," marveled Skinner. He realized after replicating the results that a basic tenet of evolutionary biology— evolution proceeds by random genetic change—had just been overturned. No longer can we view the environment as having no direct influence on the traits we pass on to our children and grandchildren. Professor Skinner speculates that his findings may help to explain the dramatic rise in breast and prostate cancer in recent decades as a reflection of the cumulative effect of various toxins over several generations.

What should also concern us are the implications these results have for our ability to rid the environment and our bodies of harm from toxic chemicals. As the publication *Rachel's Environment & Health News* described our quandary: "When persistent environmental pollutants (like DDT) are phased out, we might be falsely lulled into believing that we have solved the problem. The thinking is logical—remove the toxin from the environment and you get rid of the toxic effects. Not so according to the findings of Skinner and his colleagues. The Skinner study tells us that phasing out dangerous toxins doesn't end the problem—because the damage done by exposures decades ago could still flow from generation to generation via epigenetic pathways."

We now know how genes and the environment interact and work together. While genes may provide for a range of possible outcomes, it is the environment that determines which specific outcome is most likely to occur. Another study of toxic exposure provides us with even more evidence for this phenomenon. Blood and urine tests conducted on forty-seven female motorway tollbooth operators in Taiwan found indications of DNA damage caused by their exposure to the synergy of hundreds of pollutants in car exhaust.

How we have been treating our environment has come back to haunt us by challenging our intelligence in the most unexpected ways. Studies in Britain by Chris Williams, a social scientist at the Institute of Education at the University of London, have documented how a loss of micronutrients through soil erosion, resulting in improverished crops, combines with our exposure to synthetic chemicals to "harm the intelligence of millions of people across the world."

Our "single-substance science," says Williams, cannot account for the compounding impact of many different chemicals and environmental factors. "So the overall scale of the problem is far greater than previously estimated," he told the BBC. "The big feeling I have about this is in the context of evolution. The human brain is now at risk from its own behavior, and nothing else in the ecosystem is harming itself in the same way. We are acting like lemmings."

Harvard University biologist Stephen R. Palumbi, writing in a 2001 issue of *Science*, described how humans have created mutant bacteria, resistant to all but the most powerful antibiotics, and insects tolerant of so many different insecticides that chemical control is useless. "We are causing accelerated evolutionary changes," he concluded. It might also be added that we are altering everything, even ourselves, without having the faintest idea of the short-term, much less the long-term, implications of our actions.

An editorial in the science journal *Environmental Health Perspectives*, appearing in 1994, posed this question: "Are there specific pollutants or categories of pollutants that influence evolutionary processes? The answer to this question, based on theory and precedent, is clearly yes." An example given was the development of pesticide-resistent fish in the delta of Mississippi. These fish became genetically altered to develop a five hundredfold increase in resistance to the effects of pesticides used in agricultural areas. A commentary by a professor of toxicology noted that "studies at the cellular level have demonstrated that mutagenic chemicals can enhance the rate of development of genetically altered populations." The clear inference was left that such irreversible evolutionary changes were possible in humans as we are forced to respond to similar environmental pressures.

"You are what you eat" goes an old expression, but findings in the new science of epigenetics demonstrate that you are also what your mother ate. Epigenetics is the study of how environmental factors, such as nutrition and chemical toxins, can alter gene function without changing the DNA sequence. A mother's diet can permanently alter the functioning of genes in her offspring, concluded a 2003 study in *Molecular and Cellular Biology* that used mice to show how diet can turn genes on and off. "We have genes—including those influencing susceptibility to cancer, obesity, and diabetes—that can be turned off or on by epigenetic factors triggered by early nutrition and exposure to chemical agents," study co-author Randy Jirtle of the Duke University Department of Radiation Oncology explained to *The Wall Street Journal.*

We have seen anecdotal evidence for this phenomenon throughout history. During the Civil War and again during the Depression of the 1930s, malnourishment among pregnant women apparently resulted in a higher rate of strokes among their children and grandchildren. A similar effect was noticed in Holland in World War II when malnourishment among pregnant women apparently produced a higher-than-normal incidence of schizophrenia among their offspring.

These epigenetic effects are being described as a sort of second genetic code that is subject to the influences of toxic chemicals and nutrition.

Transcription factors is a term genetic scientists use to describe the switches that turn genes on or off. What we eat and the toxins we absorb can flip these switches and cause diseases. Massachusetts Institute of Technology scientist Rick Young predicts we will someday be able to detect transcription factor flaws in children so we can "alert parents to the fact that a change in diet might prevent development of the disease." This new field of managing our health and choosing our food based on genetic tests that isolate our personal risk factors for disease has been labeled *nutrigenomics,* the study of interactions between nutrition and genetics.

LEARNING TO PROTECT OURSELVES

Two books in 2005 tried to reassure us that the unfettered march of progress has nothing but our best interests at heart. In the first, *The Poison Paradox* by John Timbrell, a professor of biochemical toxicology at King's College London, a case was made that chemical hysteria has poisoned our minds to the many virtues of synthetic chemicals. He tells us that even when humans have contact with dioxin, one of the most poisonous of synthetic chemicals, as when an industrial accident occurred in Italy in 1976 that contaminated 17,000 people, only a few people get sick and no one dies. He explains that in theory a single molecule of some substances can cause cancer, but this is all but impossible in practice because our cells have many defenses against carcinogenic mutation. He says the likelihood of a single molecule triggering cancer is like "a single soldier destroying a military fortress." Timbrell's argument struck me as flawed because he ignores the unknown impact of toxic synergies, though I certainly agree that it is incumbent upon us to avoid the assumption that any exposure to a toxin is bound to be harmful.

The second book presents a wholly different sort of challenge. *The March of Unreason* by Lord Taverne of Pimlico, a member of the British House of Lords, amounts to a philosophical treatise arguing that organic foods, alternative medicine, and a preoccupation with toxic chemical residues are all evidence of an undercurrent of irrationality that threatens the progress and prosperity of civilization.

Since 80 percent of processed foods on supermarket shelves now contain ingredients from gene-spliced plants, and according to Lord Tav-erne, "not a single ecosystem has been disrupted" or "a person injured" by any gene-spliced product, it then follows by his logic that processed foods are superior to organic or conventionally farmed foods that use nine-teenth century or other primitive practices. Anything to the contrary, in-cluding "the widespread but baseless bias that nature knows best," is regarded by Lord Taverne as a symptom of what he describes as "eco-fundamentalism" being promulgated by shameless fear-peddlers.

On one narrow point I do find myself in agreement. Lord Taverne makes much of how U.S. government rules defining organic products are mostly nonsensical. Following certain production standards and practices does not necessarily guarantee pure products. (More on that point in the next chapter.) Yes, the regulations are highly arbitrary. Yes, under current regulations the detection of a residue of banned chemicals in foods la-beled organic doesn't violate organic standards. But to characterize as "a monument to irrationality" the entire human impulse toward organic food, based on confusing regulatory language and high product costs, is to betray the author's bias toward his own form of unreason—the mind-set that places progress at any price above any other human value, includ-ing the right to be free of chemical toxins.

We are being urged to treat all chemicals as innocent until proven guilty, even when the proof of guilt only comes when sufficient numbers of humans or animals in the wild sicken and die.The costs of such indif-ference, both to us as individuals and as a society, have become enormous. As individuals we each play Russian roulette with our health based on our daily choices about which chemicals to put in and on our bodies. As a so-ciety, out-of-control health-care costs, a direct consequence of synthetic chemicals in our food and medicine, now threaten to undermine the economy of every nation dependent upon the synthetics paradigm.

Our recent history with chemicals whose safety we were assured of il-lustrates a legitimate cause for concern. Dozens of examples exist. Here are just two of them.

A synthetic estrogen, DES, manufactured from coal tar derivatives, was introduced to treat menopausal women in the United States and Eu-rope under several hundred brand names in the 1940s. No human clinical trials were done, but animal testing found no health danger. Millions of pregnant women also were encouraged to take this wonder drug because, as one drug company declared in its 1957 advertising campaign, DES "produces bigger and stronger babies." Starting in 1947, beef cattle were also fed DES as a growth stimulant; later it became a feed additive for fattening chickens and other livestock.

After nearly three decades of use the horrific discovery was made that DES was causing spontaneous abortions, premature births, and neonatal deaths. In pregnant women DES crossed the placenta into their fetuses and disrupted fetal development, or hid in the female children's bodies until later in life when it caused vaginal cancer.

As a second illustration consider what happened with DDT. It was introduced as a bug killer following World War II, and its effectiveness as a pesticide was hailed as another modern miracle for human health and the conveniences of life. You may have seen that famous photograph of children playing happily in the spray of a DDT truck that's fogging mosquitoes. Not until Rachel Carson's 1962 book, *Silent Spring*, did we come to understand the serious reproductive health problems that DDT was inflicting on wildlife, or the disastrous potential for harm it posed to humans as an endocrine disrupter of the first order.

Protecting ourselves from what we don't know can harm us sometimes requires a leap of faith into self-reliance. When authority figures and institutions fail us, when the resulting apocalyptic scenarios challenge our ability to cope, we have five thousand years of ancient wisdom about food and medicine to fall back upon.

PART THREE

BEYOND APOCALYPSE NOW

Our Natural Legacy

We can harness the power of positive, health-enhancing synergies from foods and herbs to strengthen our immune systems. Using food as medicine enables us to detoxify ourselves of chemical contaminants and cure ourselves of illness and disease.

An ancient legacy of naturally occurring health and healing is based on thousands of years of human experience with wisdom traditions that follow the principles of nature. These natural cures are being affirmed by Western medicine in laboratory experiments that show them to be more effective, less costly, and less toxic than most pharmaceutical drugs.

CHAPTER SEVEN

OUR HEALTH IS NATURALLY OCCURRING

"Nature distributed medicine everywhere."

—Pliny the Elder

"The aim of medicine is to prevent disease and prolong life; the ideal of medicine is to eliminate the need of a physician."

—William J. Mayo, founder of the Mayo Clinic

Nothing in his training could have prepared Mark J. Plotkin for what he witnessed in the Amazon jungle when a tribal shaman administered an effective herbal cure for severe diabetes to a dying woman. It was a cure that Western medical science cannot duplicate. Seeing the evidence of a natural healing synergy having been evoked by an ancient wisdom tradition contradicted most everything Plotkin had learned about medicine as a Harvard- and Yale-educated ethnobotanist, and as a Ph.D. research associate with the Smithsonian Institution's Museum of Natural History.

The patient was a thirty-five-year-old woman of the Tirio Indian tribe who was stretched out on a cot in a village hut, dying of type 2 diabetes. A physician accompanying Plotkin had measured her blood sugar at a near-fatal level. Short of shooting her full of insulin, there was nothing this Western-trained physician or Plotkin could do for her.

At this point a shaman healer from a neighboring tribe arrived with a potion he said would cure the patient. The potion was a thick reddish-brown liquid that had been concocted by combining the inner bark of a particular type of tree with crushed leaves of herbs and the sap of a gray vine, all boiled together over a wood fire. The shaman administered two spoons of the oral remedy to the woman and continued this treatment four times a day.

Plotkin describes what happened next in his 2000 book, *Medicine Quest*: "Within three days, she felt well enough to return to working in her garden, something she'd been unable to do for two years. By the end of the week, her blood-sugar level was normal."

Here the story took an even more perplexing turn for Plotkin when he took samples of the ingredients used in the shaman's diabetes cure back to the United States and had them analyzed by chemists in a laboratory. The test results turned out negative—at least by standards of Western medical science—for any active healing properties that could be isolated in the separate compounds.

"Meanwhile," relates Plotkin, "three women in the village who had been certified as diabetics by a visiting physician continued to enjoy robust health while taking the shaman's potion. Puzzled and frustrated, I asked a chemist who had worked on the analysis if he could explain the discrepancy between what I was seeing in the field and what was happening (or not happening) in the laboratory. He noted that lab analysis often consists of an initial search for the 'therapeutically active compounds'— the chemicals powerful enough to account for the action of the potion— and then the testing of each component separately."

"Shamanistic medicine often depends on synergy," continues Plotkin, "how the chemical components of the herbs interact with each other, or how the shaman's practices—chanting, aromatherapy, or massage, in some cases—create a mental state that interacts with the plant chemicals." In other words, the combination of synergistic principles, some involving chemistry, some the mind/body interactions that are described in Western medicine as the placebo effect, account for these seemingly miraculous herbal cures in the jungle.

This was precisely what the shaman had told Plotkin: "I make the potion from four plants and *every* plant in the potion contributes to the healing process. Do you think I would waste my time adding useless plants to my medicine?"

Western medicine's obsession with magic bullets, attempting to isolate single active molecules as healing triggers, misses an entire range of extraordinary therapeutic gifts available in nature. The applications of synergistic principles for healing by so-called primitive cultures have been ignored or treated with ridicule. Plotkin is now a scientist who can testify from firsthand knowledge how modern chemistry and technology can only supplement—not replace—the wisdom of nature.

"The future of Western healing," he declares, "is complementary medicine, which brings together the best of all healing traditions under one roof: from acupuncture to shamanistic hypnotherapy to surgery. And natural products—herbs, vitamins, and other supplements—will prove to be an integral part of this new healing tradition."

Former Harvard Botanical Museum researcher Andrew Weil laments how in the West "science and medicine have separated themselves from nature and separated us from nature." Healing is a natural process, "and if you want to understand healing and how to make people better, you must understand the ways of nature. The message that's not overtly stated but is between the lines [of modern Western medicine] is that nature is fundamentally wild, dangerous, and unpredictable. It's out to get you, whereas the products of pharmaceutical laboratories are safe. That message is especially annoying because it's actually the other way around, and I say that as a doctor who often has to deal with the casualties of pharmaceutical science."

Mother Nature has been creating and perfecting healing chemicals in plants for nearly four billion years. We have only to watch animals in the wild, such as chimpanzees, and note how they select plants to prevent and treat illness, to understand their intuitive grasp of nature's pharmaceutical potential. When plants used by animals for medicine are analyzed, humans invariably discover they possess antibacterial and antiparasitic qualities. Instead of trying to find a single active ingredient inside a single plant, as drug laboratories do, animals and the tribal societies that watch and learn from animal behaviors utilize the entire plant and its dozens of compounds, often mixed with other plants. Both in tribal wisdom and in animal instinctive wisdom there is an understanding that the healing comes from the resulting synergy.

Naturally occurring synergies are a principle in all aspects of nature and in our human nature as well. Synergies occur at every step in the process of our experience of food. To bake a particular type of cake, for instance, specific ingredients are required—eggs, sugar, salt, flour, etc.—which must be mixed and exposed to heat for the varied ingredients to produce a specific taste. What our taste buds respond to are the combined synergistic effects of this process. Similarly, when we digest the cake, digestive synergies occur within our stomachs and intestines that determine whether our body will metabolize or reject the meal.

"The human immune system is another miracle of synergy," writes biologist Peter Corning in *Nature's Magic.* "The highly evolved system that defends our bodies against the enormous number of potentially harmful microbes in our environment consists of nine different 'sub-systems' . . . these highly specialized parts can do things that none of them could do alone. It's a synergistic system."

We see the principle of synergy at work in our lives in both positive and negative ways. At the heart of the polymer chemistry field, which has given us synthetic rubber and fibers and plastics, are synergistic principles that produce elasticity, toughness, and other valued qualities for products. Negative synergy, sometimes referred to as *dysergy,* displays its most toxic effects in the realm of human biochemistry and health. We have seen in earlier chapters how synthetic chemicals combine into toxic synergies within our foods, our medicines, and our environment to harm human health and reproduction.

Synergistic principles used by traditional medicine from China and India don't target herbs for a given disease or malady, as happens with the magic bullet approach of Western pharmaceutical companies. Instead, a mixture of herbs is designed to energize and stimulate the entire body while facilitating the immune system to do its job more effectively. An example of a natural synergy harnessed to combat a major disease is Carctol, a mixture of eight medicinal herbs from traditional Hindu medicine that is being used to help people rid themselves of cancer. A study of 1,900 Indian cancer patients who took the mixture found that 75 percent experienced benefits, defined as more energy, weight gain, calmness, and tumor shrinkage.

Pharmacist Ross Pelton, co-author of *Mind Food and Smart Pills*, describes an ancient Chinese treatise on medicinal herbs, dating back to 2700 BC, that gives 365 herbs, and their health uses, which are still being applied today. "A particular herb may contain several active ingredients that increase each other's effects. In some herbal blends secondary herbs are added to support the absorption, transport, and effectiveness of the primary herb. Each is integral for the effectiveness of the other."

Our health is naturally occurring and was intended to be maintained by the natural synergies generated by essential nutrients found in our foods. We are amazing biochemical marvels of nature, possessing ingenious immune systems designed to keep us healthy by repelling toxic invaders and repairing damage caused by the wear of age and living. Herbs and other products of nature support our immune systems when they are needed. But this entire strategy for a healthy life is dependent on what we do and don't put into our bodies.

PURE FOOD IS GOOD MEDICINE

For half of the twentieth century Henry G. Bieler was known as the "physician to the stars," treating legendary actresses Gloria Swanson and Greta Garbo and other celebrities among his stable of devoted patients. What attracted this famous clientele was also what set Bieler apart from other physicians of his day—a philosophy emphasizing how "food, not drugs, is your best medicine."

Medicine's founding father, Hippocrates of ancient Greece, in one of his many quotable aphorisms observed how, "Nature heals; the physician is only nature's assistant." Bieler took that advice as his inspiration to "rediscover some ancient truths" and apply them to medicine. The first truth: Hippocrates had prescribed treating illness first by a diet regimen, second with medicines, and lastly with surgery. Modern physicians had reversed the order of treatments and Bieler made it his mission to reinstate the ancient value system.

"This is the Dark Age of medicine," declared Dr. Bieler, citing Western medicine's obsession with prescription drugs and its refusal to accept that "nature does the real healing, utilizing the natural defenses of the body."

Far in advance of his time, Bieler came to a series of intuitive and commonsense conclusions that we are now reaffirming through trial and error: using drugs for treatment is often harmful, causing serious side effects; most illness "can be cured through the proper use of correct foods" and periods of fasting to detoxify the body; the buildup of chemical toxins in the body causes disease; we have become so preoccupied with synthesizing chemicals in the laboratory that "we have lost sight of the fact that these same chemicals have been lodged in our foods for many thousands of years"; the use of synthetic vitamins does nothing for human health and depletes our financial resources while "lining the pockets of the pharmaceutical houses"; and the processed foods that people consume today are "about as far removed from the natural diet of man as man is from his primitive jungle . . . [but man] still has approximately the same digestive apparatus and liver as his remote ancestors."

Instead of "stuffing the sick with powerful toxic drugs and then other drugs to 'remedy the remedy,' " as other physicians did, Bieler would have his patients fast on vegetable broths or diluted fruit juices "to give the exhausted body organs an opportunity to discharge their waste products and heal themselves." He decried how "anxiety-ridden Americans" had fallen prey to the advertising of processed foods companies and pharmaceutical companies to "consider health something that can be purchased in a bottle at the drugstore." In so doing they forgot, if they ever knew, "that health can be found only by obeying the clear-cut laws of nature."

Bieler's insights have been affirmed and expanded by Jean Carper, author of such books as *Food: Your Miracle Medicine* and *The Food Pharmacy.* Carper rooted her books in the findings of more than ten thousand medical studies she analyzed and contrasted, all excavated from the databases of the National Library of Medicine in Bethesda, Maryland, and the University of Illinois at Chicago, which maintains huge medical resources on the pharmacological properties of foods and plants.

"Food is the breakthrough drug of the twenty-first century," Carper concluded. "Despite our man-made wonder drugs, Mother Nature is truly the world's oldest and greatest pharmacist. Mainstream scientists are increasingly reaching back to the truths of ancient food folk medicine and dietary practices."

Foods can induce a range of therapeutic effects on human body functions, acting as anticoagulants, analgesics, sedatives, cholesterol reducers, cancer fighters, immune stimulators, anti-inflammatories, and on and on. The medicinal effects of food are synergistic. "A single food contains hundreds or thousands of chemicals, most unidentified, that make up each bite's pharmacological activity," says Carper.

A similar point was made in a 2001 issue of the *Townsend Letter for Doctors and Patients*: "Whole food, grown on organic, nutrient-rich and chemical-free soil in a clean environment, provides the body with a synergistic array of thousands of known and unknown antioxidants, nutrients, and powerful nutraceutical compounds."

Just for good measure, let's refer to several more experts on nutrition who understand the synergistic principles at work in food. "Every vegetable, every fruit, has literally hundreds of constituents—any protection is likely due to a combination rather than a single chemical," observes Lee Wattenberg, an authority on human enzymes at the University of Minnesota. Marion Nestle, professor of nutrition at New York University, speaking to *The New York Times*, adds: "The evidence is pretty clear that foods work [in promoting health], but single nutrients don't."

Finally, we have this perspective from T. Colin Campbell, professor emeritus of nutritional biochemistry at Cornell University, who co-conducted a comprehensive study of nutrition in China that was published as a book in 2005. He identified some important principles linking nutrition and health: (1) Nutrition represents the combined activities of countless food substances, and the whole truly is greater than the sum of its parts. (2) Genes don't determine diseases on their own but are activated or expressed as a result of nutrition. (3) Nutrition can substantially control the adverse effects of toxic chemicals that we ingest or absorb.

"There is enough evidence now that doctors should be discussing the option of pursuing dietary change as a potential path to cancer prevention and treatment," writes Campbell. "A whole-foods, plant-based diet may be an incredibly effective anti-cancer medicine."

THE MEDICINAL WONDER FOODS

At least five thousand years ago the stinky white bulb we call garlic was being pounded into medicinal foods to ward off illness and disease. One builder of an Egyptian pyramid even carved into the monument an account of how much garlic his work crews consumed to stay healthy.

As one of humanity's earliest healers, garlic was prized because it produced noticeable effects in strengthening immunity. It was no coincidence that in Dracula legend and lore the cloves of garlic provided immunity against the vampire's attempts to drain a person's lifeblood.

We have rediscovered this ancient wisdom about garlic in modern laboratory settings. Over the past few decades about one thousand science articles have appeared touting the medicinal properties of this pungent root. Garlic contains up to two hundred compounds and active ingredients, including selenium, sulfur compounds, potassium, phosphorus, amino acids, vitamins B and C, copper, and zinc. While there is evidence for the health effects of single ingredients, what makes garlic so potent for overall human health is the synergistic effect of all these natural chemicals working together.

At the molecular level, experiments have demonstrated specific ways that garlic activates the immune system. "[Our findings] do substantiate that garlic widens blood vessels and reduces hypertension," observed the leader of one experiment, David Julius, a professor in the department of cellular and molecular pharmacology at the University of California at San Francisco.

Other scientists have shown how allicin, a substance garlic excretes when squeezed, is a natural antibiotic that kills bacteria and intestinal parasites. Experiments on laboratory animals at Pennsylvania State University discovered how garlic powder protects against breast cancer, while physicians at UCLA uncovered evidence that garlic stops a variety of cancers from growing. Studies in *Annals of Internal Medicine* (1993) and the *Journal of Physiology and Pharmacology* (1979) both found persuasive evidence that garlic significantly decreases cholesterol levels in most people.

Broccoli is another powerful ally for the human immune system. A study by a research team at Johns Hopkins University published in a 2005 issue of *Proceedings of the National Academy of Sciences* uncovered strong evidence that phytochemicals in broccoli detoxify certain cancer-causing agents and also act in producing enzymes that fight pain and inflammation, making broccoli potentially more effective than Vioxx and other prescription drugs commonly issued for arthritic conditions.

Almost every major medical condition is either caused by or affected by what you eat, says Isadore Rosenfeld. "Yet very few medical doctors are knowledgeable about nutrition. As a result, they rarely give nutritional advice—even when specific foods can help curb symptoms or correct underlying problems as well as or better than prescription medications."

Nutritionists and physicians who have taken the time to study nutrient values generally recommend these natural foods for health: Mushrooms are high in B vitamins and selenium, and studies have shown they boost immune system activity, elevate antioxidants, and lower blood pressure and insulin levels. Blueberries and spinach are both high in vitamins and antioxidants. Walnuts, Brazil nuts, and almonds are immune system boosters from the nut family. Most of the cruciferous vegetables—broccoli, cabbage, cauliflower, collard greens, turnips, kale, and radishes—have demonstrated their effectiveness against colon cancer and intestinal polyps.

When fruits and vegetables are analyzed for their antioxidant potential, a score known as oxygen radical absorbance capacity, five foods in each category stand out for their health benefits: among fruits, prunes score 5,770, raisins 2,830, blueberries 2,400, blackberries 2,036, and strawberries 1,540; among vegetables, kale scores 1,770, spinach 1,260, brussels sprouts 980, alfalfa sprouts 930, and broccoli 890.

MYTHS WE CHERISH

ONLY DRUGS CAN TREAT DEPRESSION

An estimated nineteen million Americans have been diagnosed with depression and treated with pharmaceutical drugs, a number that represents, as a percentage of the total population, an increase of more than 300 percent since World War II. Even if we take into account higher stress associated with changes in lifestyle and work habits over a half century, common sense tells us that something else must be contributing to this upsurge of mood disorders that we see manifested in depression, behavioral and attention problems among children, and antisocial criminal behaviors among teenagers.

Carbohydrate cravings, unexplained weight gain, and fatigue are some of the symptoms associated with a disorder known as atypical depression, which afflicts nearly half of all people diagnosed with depression. A study published in the *Journal of Psychiatric Practice* during 2005 found a direct link between this form of depression and a deficiency of essential nutrients in diet.

A randomized, double-blind study of 113 people—eighteen to sixty-five years old—with atypical depression found those exhibiting the most intense symptoms tested positive for a chromium deficiency. Those patients in the eight-week study given a chromium picolinate supplement showed "significantly greater improvements" in all symptoms related to their depression. Chromium is a trace mineral in food and is essential to enabling us to metabolize carbohydrates, fats, and proteins. It works as a preventive against diabetes. Normally it would be found in our soils and in foods like whole grains, onions, lettuce, and tomatoes, but depletion of soil nutrients and food processing has taken most of it out of our diet.

"For years, the link between depression, insulin sensitivity, and the value of dietary chromium picolinate has been hinted at in small studies," declared lead investigator John Docherty, a professor of psychiatry at Cornell University.

Contained within this study we find a revelation that is a smoking-gun indictment of pharmaceutical drug treatments of atypical depression. "The use of antidepressants, mood stabilizers, and antipsychotics that are commonly prescribed to treat depression can often worsen carbohydrate cravings," revealed Docherty. Other nutritional researchers have pointed out that prescription drugs routinely deplete stores of essential minerals in the body, such as chromium.

These findings strongly suggest that the synthetic drugs millions of people routinely take for depression may be aggravating the underlying cause of their depression. In other words, your cure may be doing more long-term harm than good, while the real cure is the return to a naturally occurring substance that has been depleted from your diet.

Still another link between a naturally occurring substance and depression comes from a massive study of pregnant women in Britain. More than fourteen thousand expectant mothers were recruited, and then the women and their children were monitored for eleven years by the University of Bristol and other collaborators for information about eating habits, experiences of violence, stress, mood disorders, etc.

A major finding was a fiftyfold greater rate of major depression among those women who had the lowest levels of seafood consumption. This finding mirrored results of postnatal surveys from twenty-three countries that found depression occurs less frequently in those countries, like Japan, with high seafood consumption.

The substance in seafood that turned out to be responsible for providing protection against depression was omega-3 essential fatty acids, which cannot be made by the human body and are necessary for the membranes of neurons in the brain. A United States Public Health Service official, Joseph Hibbeln, describes how omega-3s have been replaced in our diet by the less-healthy omega-6 fatty acids from seed oils: "During the four to five million years of human evolution the dietary ratio of omega-6 fatty acids to omega-3 fatty acids was approximately 1:1. However, the omega-3 family (found in fish, seafood, walnuts, leafy vegetables) is getting pushed out of the brain by a huge rise in intake of omega-6 (from meat, corn oil, soybean oil, and other oils). The ratio is now estimated to be in the region of 15:1. Increasing prevalence rates of major depression in the United States are closely correlated to the increasing amounts of omega-6 fatty acids in the food supply."

As the consumption of omega-3s fell and the intake of omega-6s rose, Hibbeln has documented, a corresponding escalation occurred in the homicide rates of the twenty-six countries studied where statistics for homicides and seafood consumption are kept. A lifetime of nutritional deficiencies can result in a lifetime of depression or criminal behavior.

To avoid coming down with depression or seasonal affective disorder, which impacts an estimated 17 percent of all U.S. residents over the course of a lifetime, experts recommend omega-3 supplements, the herb called Saint-John's-wort, and the synergistic effects of a healthy, pure-foods diet. "The foundation of a depression-free lifestyle consists of a good diet, a regular exercise and stress-reduction program, and elimination of all chemical addictions," says Hyla Cass, assistant clinical professor of psychiatry at the UCLA School of Medicine.

MYTHS WE CHERISH
FOOD DOESN'T CAUSE VIOLENCE

"You do what you eat" might be a new slogan for the emerging evidence that a solution to violent thoughts and criminal behaviors may be in our dining habits and on our plates every day.

A large-scale study—its results published in 2002 in *The British Journal of Psychiatry*—used 231 young adult prisoners, ages eighteen to twenty-one, to test the idea that supplements containing vitamins, minerals, and essential fatty acids could reduce the incidence of violence. The supplements included omega-3 fatty acids, chromium, and two dozen other vitamins and minerals. Prisoners remained on this regimen for 142 days, and their number of disciplinary incidents was compared over this period to a control group of inmates.

Compared to the baseline group, the supplement takers recorded a 37 percent drop in the number of serious disruptive incidents, including violence. It was powerful evidence that poor nutrition plays a key role in triggering violent and antisocial aggressive behavior. "Most criminal justice systems assume that criminal behavior is entirely a matter of free will," observes study author C. Bernard Gesch, a senior research scientist in physiology at the University of Oxford. "But how exactly can you exercise free will without involving your brain? How exactly can the brain function without an adequate nutrient supply? I think nutrition may actually be one of the most straightforward factors to change antisocial behavior. It's also cheap and humane."

Our brains are metabolic engines that take up just 2 percent of our body mass and yet use 20 percent of the nutrients we burn. It stands to reason that if the brain's requirement for essential nutrients from food sources isn't met, there will be mood and behavioral consequences.

In a presentation before members of the British Parliament in 2003, Gesch described how crime statistics for England and Wales showed a tenfold increase since the 1950s, not coincidentally the very period when the essential nutrient content of fruits and vegetables underwent a precipitous decline. For example, in 1946 the biggest source of vitamin C was fresh vegetables, but by 1993 the primary source had become fizzy drinks laden with chemical additives. Criminal statistics for the United States paint an even bleaker picture. As of the summer of 2005, nearly ten thousand U.S. prison inmates were serving life sentences for murder and other violent crimes they committed before the age of 18, a total more than all of the other industrialized nations combined.

Many previous studies support Gesch's findings. In the United States an experimental study of three thousand imprisoned juveniles in 1983 replaced snack foods with a range of healthier options. Over the next year there followed a 21 percent reduction in antisocial behaviors, a 100 percent reduction in suicides, and a 25 percent reduction in assaults. The creator of this experiment, Stephen Schoenthaler of California State University, is considered a pioneer in showing the relationships between nutrition and behavior, especially criminal behavior. He has also published papers in *The Lancet* and other medical journals demonstrating how vitamin and mineral supplementation can improve children's intelligence and school performance.

Other studies have produced evidence that zinc deficiencies in diet can contribute to criminal behaviors among juveniles because zinc is important to making chemical transmitters in the brain. "We think that it is a direct result of exposure to chemical toxins . . . which prevent the absorption of zinc," declares Neil Ward, senior lecturer in analytical chemistry at Britain's Surrey University.

Gesch sees a theme in all of these findings—healthy food can create a healthier society. "Is it plausible that in the last fifty years we could have made spectacular changes to the human diet without any implications for the brain? I don't think so. Now, evidence is mounting that putting poor fuel into the brain significantly affects social behavior. We need to know more about the composition of the right nutrients. It could be the recipe for peace."

MYTHS WE CHERISH

ONLY DRUGS CAN RELIEVE PAIN

Chronic or recurrent pain afflicts an estimated one in six persons in the United States and costs the nation at least $100 billion a year in lost productivity and health-care costs. A major reason most of these people fail to find pain relief, according to a cover story in *Time* magazine (February 28, 2005), is that "most of us seek it entirely in a pill bottle—or two or three."

What we miss by fixating on pharmaceutical drugs is an entire arsenal of pain fighters that are naturally occurring and have no toxic side effects. White willow bark and bromelain are two natural substances with demonstrated pain-relief potential that work quickly and without the side effects seen in prescription or over-the-counter synthetics.

Ethnobotanist Mark J. Plotkin identifies a range of natural drugs that are now in the pipeline for development as painkillers. These range from cone snails, snake venom, and frog skin poison to a host of marine organisms and even soil fungi with high antibiotic properties. "There are certain things that Western medicine cannot do well, and relieving pain naturally is one of them," says Plotkin.

At the University of California at Davis counselors in the pain management center teach patients how to relieve pain symptoms using guided imagery, deep breathing, yoga, meditation, hypnotherapy, acupuncture, and other natural distraction techniques. "Learning to relieve fear, anxiety, and depression related to pain actually helps bring relief, probably by activating the body's own pain-killing chemicals," Scott Fishman, chief of pain medicine at UC Davis, told a *Time* magazine interviewer.

Positive thinking can be as powerful as a shot of morphine in relieving pain, a team of Wake Forest University researchers has found. By using functional magnetic resonance imaging (MRI) on ten volunteers, they discovered that areas of the brain important to pain processing had decreased activity when the volunteers lowered their expectations of experiencing pain. They simply put their attention on the belief that pain would not feel as severe as they would normally experience it. "Pain needs to be treated with more than just pills," commented Robert Coghill, who led the research team, which published their findings in a 2005 issue of *Proceedings of the National Academy of Sciences.*

An even more astonishing method of relieving pain naturally comes from research at the Lister Hospital in London, described in a 2005 article in *New Scientist.* A forty-six-year-old woman was hypnotized and underwent breast surgery without general anesthesia. Afterward she proclaimed, "The plastic surgeon was cutting and sewing inside me, but I couldn't feel any sensation at all." Unlike her previous experiences with painkillers, she experienced no nausea or other side effects from hypnosis.

An estimated five thousand surgical procedures using hypnosis as a pain reliever have been carried out at Liege Hospital in Belgium. The primary benefit of this non-drug approach—other than fewer side effects—has been less bleeding during surgery. Anesthetic drugs inhibit the natural ability of blood vessels to constrict when incisions are made into the body, while hypnosis enables the vessels to constrict and reduce blood loss.

At the University of Florida, medical researchers taught women self-hypnosis techniques to use before giving birth. These women required significantly less medication, had fewer complications during delivery, and generally delivered healthier babies than women who used prescription drugs. No one is sure yet just how or why hypnosis works in relieving or eliminating pain, but somehow signals are blocked in those areas of the brain that perceive pain.

MYTHS WE CHERISH

PLACEBOS DON'T REALLY HEAL

Whenever we hear the word *placebo* it's usually in association with a double-blind clinical trial study of some new pharmaceutical drug. We sometimes learn at the end of the study if the drug did or didn't surpass the placebo in its effectiveness at relieving the symptoms of an ailment or disease.

What few people bother to investigate further is whether the placebo, from Latin for "I will please," stands on its own as a naturally occurring process for healing that any one of us can use in our life, without help from a physician or the need to participate in a clinical drug trial.

Placebos are quite simply those beliefs that enable our mind to interact with our immune system to create a healing synergy. A placebo is the most naturally occurring and powerful process of physical and mental health that we possess.

"Medicine is woven into the stuff of the mind," said Hippocrates more than 2,500 years ago. Today we are rediscovering this ancient wisdom as evidence of "mind over matter" medicine emerges from experiments addressing a wide range of health concerns.

"Hundreds of experiments show that psychological factors—things in the mind—affect the body, including the immune system—the molecules and cells we mobilize to fight off illness," wrote Melvin Konner in his 1993 book, *Medicine at the Crossroads.*

A pioneering study documenting how powerful the placebo effect can be appeared in a 1959 issue of *The New England Journal of Medicine* describing fake operations. Cardiology patients who got fake operations for angina pain experienced as much benefit as patients who actually had the surgery to tie off their arteries. "They experienced reduction of pain, took fewer nitroglycerin tablets to control their angina, resumed normal activity, and even had improvements in their electrocardiogram tracings—all to the same extent as those who got the full operation," marveled Konner.

Harvard Medical School professor Jerry Avorn describes in his book *Powerful Medicines* how a placebo can be just as effective as synthetic drugs, with many fewer side effects. "A pivotal paper published in the British journal *The Lancet* in 1978 placed the once touchy-feely placebo effect firmly in the realm of hard-science neuropharmacology. The study started out as a typical pain experiment: volunteers were given an inert placebo and, as expected, a substantial proportion of them reported that it reduced their pain. But when these subjects were given the opioid blocker naloxone, it blocked the placebo benefit as well. This suggested that the placebo effect results in part from a person's capacity to secrete homemade narcotics within the brain itself." Avorn says the proven benefits of the placebo give "new meaning to the once-dismissive phrase, 'It's all in your head.' "

Here is just a sampling of the range of medical evidence emerging for the healing powers of placebos:

• Detailed scans of brains cells in Parkinson's disease patients revealed that patients who received placebos (in the form of a salt solution) responded in the same way and with the same level of relief as they would in receiving a drug to relieve their symptoms. This study, performed at the University of Turin Medical School in Italy, discovered that the placebo effect caused a release of dopamine, a lack of which causes Parkinson's patients' tremors and muscle rigidity. (Published in *Nature Neuroscience*, 2004.)

- People who suffer from depression and receive a placebo not only usually improve, but a section of their brain linked to memory and attention becomes activated; this same brain area is repressed as a side effect when the patients take antidepressant drugs. "People who get better on placebo have a change in brain function just as surely as people who get better on medication," said Andrew Leuchter of the University of California at Los Angeles, who led the nine-week study of fifty-one patients. "We now know that placebo is very definitely an active treatment condition." (Published in *The American Journal of Psychiatry*, 2001.)

- In a remarkable demonstration of how positive thoughts strengthen your immune system while negative thoughts can make you ill, researchers from the University of Wisconsin–Madison studied fifty-two people ranging in age between fifty-seven and sixty and measured their brain activity as they thought of past events that made them happy, sad, afraid, or angry. Afterward each volunteer was given a flu vaccine shot. Over the next six months each volunteer was tested to measure the level of antibodies generated by the vaccine. Those who had previously shown the most powerful activity in the right prefrontal cortex of the brain—an area pessimists show more activity in—had the worst immune system reactions to the flu shot, while people with the most healthy reaction to the shot were those who had their most powerful brain reactions in the left prefrontal cortex, the side associated with optimists. (Published in *Proceedings of the National Academy of Sciences*, 2005.)

Though the field of psychoneuroimmunology—the study of the brain's interaction with the immune system—is only a few decades old, physicians no longer have any excuse to be unaware of it. The mass of scientific evidence supporting the placebo's usefulness as a natural healing mechanism has grown too large for competent health-care workers to overlook. Yet, even those who use placebos in their practice still seem almost ashamed of them.

A 2004 study in the *British Medical Journal* revealed that three of every five doctors in Jerusalem routinely give patients placebos out of a curiosity about their effectiveness. An astounding 94 percent of the physicians and nurses surveyed said sugar pills were effective in relieving symptoms ranging from asthma to angina and vertigo. (Perhaps there is shame attached when placebos raise an ethical issue—doctors prescribing sugar pill placebos and charging patients the prescription drug rates.)

Harvard Medical School professor Herbert Benson has been a pioneer in exploring and explaining how our mind affects the body to facilitate healing. In his 1997 book, *Timeless Healing,* he describes how each of us has a "remembered wellness" and "in large measure, the history of medicine is the history of the placebo effect." He bemoans how "physicians just don't understand the placebo effect, still considering the placebo a scientific anomaly or unscientific." But Benson is an optimist at heart, confessing that "we are, without a doubt, at a turning point in the history of belief in healing. Clearly the public is ahead of medicine in articulating the void."

MYTHS WE CHERISH

ORGANIC FOOD IS ALWAYS PURE

Many of us have understandably chosen to believe that any food bearing the label "organic" is automatically superior. We believe *organic* denotes a pure food that is free of pesticides and synthetic chemical additives and that it has been declared truly organic by some impartial authority. But our trust has sometimes been misplaced.

Ever since 1940, when a British scientist, Sir Albert Howard, laid down the theoretical foundation of organic farming, a basic tenet of organic philosophy has been that crops must grow free of synthetic chemicals to maintain high levels of nutrients. It is believed that herbicides, pesticides, and fast-acting, inorganic fertilizers destroy or disrupt essential microbiotic activity in the soil, thus further diminishing nutrients and food flavor.

Proponents of industrial agriculture seem to take delight in pointing out that testing of organic produce still turns up small pesticide residues, no matter how rigorous or pure the production standards. Why do organic products made without synthetic chemicals still contain them?

A 2002 study appearing in the peer-reviewed journal *Food Additives and Contaminants* revealed three reasons for pesticide residues on organic foods: (1) Past pesticide use leaves soil contaminated through successive growing seasons. (2) Wind carries pesticide sprays from nearby nonorganic farms. (3) Some tested samples have been mislabeled as organic, either due to innocent mistakes or fraud.

Since 1990 many of the corporate giants of food processing, such as General Mills, Heinz, Dole, Kraft, Gerber, ConAgra, and Archer Daniels Midland, have either acquired or created organic product brands. Much like what happened when the vitamin industry came to be dominated by pharmaceutical companies, this takeover of organic foods by the makers of chemical foods threatens to water down or degrade organic standards, until the word itself becomes just another meaningless marketing term.

The latest evidence comes from attempts in late 2005 by Dole, Kraft, and the other major players in organic foods to amend the national organic standards regulations enforced by the United States Department of Agriculture so that hundreds of synthetic substances used in conventional food processing could be used in the production of organic foods. These synthetic chemicals include leavening agents, ripening agents, thickeners, and a range of other ingredients.

Previous attempts to weaken the definition of *organic* were even more flagrantly absurd. In 1997 and 1998 the USDA, prodded by industry, proposed that genetic engineering, food irradiation, and even the use of toxic sewage sludge be permissible for use on organic farms, while in 2004 the USDA tried to allow pesticides and antibiotics to fall under the label of organic. Each time, an outcry from organic foods consumers forced the government and large corporate producers to back down.

Despite these ongoing attempts to undermine organic standard, research has shown that organic fruits and vegetables contain only about one-third of the number of chemical residues found on conventionally grown foods. The levels of contamination for each type of chemical residue also test much lower in the organic foods.

What continues to set organic foods clearly apart from foods intentionally doused with chemicals are the nutritional advantages. A study in the *Journal of Applied Nutrition* analyzed and contrasted the mineral content of conventionally grown versus organically grown potatoes, pears, apples, sweet corn, and wheat over a two-year period. Organic proved far higher in mineral content by these percentages: selenium, 390 percent; magnesium, 138 percent; potassium, 125 percent; chromium, 78 percent; iodine, 73 percent; calcium, 63 percent; zinc, 60 percent; iron, 59 percent.

Another study, this one from the University of California at Davis, found that organic berries and corn carry 50 percent higher levels of phenolic compounds—antioxidants believed to reduce the risk of heart disease and cancer—than do conventionally grown berries and corn. A reason why came from Alyson E. Mitchell, an assistant professor of food chemistry who led the study: Since phenols are generated in response to attacks by fungus or insects, plants not being defended by pesticides produce them in abundance.

A Scottish biochemist, John Paterson, trumpets still another health advantage of organics. Research studies have shown that soup made from organic vegetables contains six times the levels of salicylic acid found in nonorganic vegetable soup. Salicylic acid is the active anti-inflammatory ingredient in aspirin, and evidence suggests that it can reduce the risk for heart disease and bowel cancer.

Considering all of these scientifically demonstrated health benefits from organic foods, one might hope and trust that the standards for organic would be strengthened, or at least maintained at reasonably high levels, and not be diluted by the economic impulse for quick fixes and profit considerations. If current trends provide any indication, our hopes in this regard will rest with vigilant consumers of organic products.

MYTHS WE CHERISH
CENTENARIANS ARE GENETIC ANOMALIES

You may have heard the stories of the 112-year-old woman who still smokes cigars and drinks moonshine whiskey, or the 110-year-old man who attributes his longevity to feasting on pork rinds and chasing wild women. There are a few genetic anomalies out there, people who can spend a lifetime making food and lifestyle choices that would victimize most of the rest of us with illness, disease, depression, and a shortened life.

Yet, the more people who live to one hundred years of age and beyond are studied, the more we learn how small a role genetic programming in and of itself plays in extending life spans. A report cosponsored by the American Association of Retired Persons estimated that genes account for only 30 percent of longevity in humans, with the remainder determined by diet and lifestyle factors.

Scattered around the planet are communities of people for whom living to one hundred—and doing so in a state of good health—is considered normal and expected. Two pockets of longevity in particular, the Hunzas of Pakistan and the Okinawans of Japan, offer us clues about how to achieve our own naturally occurring states of health with extended age.

The Hunza people live in a remote valley of far northeastern Pakistan, completely enclosed by mountain peaks. They are less than fifty thousand in number, and their average age at death is at least ninety, compared with seventy-seven in the United States. What impresses visitors more than their long lives is how vigorous and healthy they normally remain right up until death.

American cardiologists Paul White and Edward Toomey conducted a medical study of twenty-five Hunza men between the ages of ninety and 110 and discovered that not a single one of them displayed any signs of high cholesterol, high blood pressure, or coronary artery disease. Optometrist Allen Banik studied the eyes of the oldest Hunza and pronounced them "to be perfect." He later wrote about his findings in a book, declaring "everything that I had read about perpetual life and health in this tiny country is true."

The Hunzas' farming methods are entirely organic, and processed foods and synthetic chemicals are foreign to their experience. Most food is eaten raw, and during the late spring the people traditionally engage in fasting before the new harvest becomes available. All children are breast-fed, birth defects are almost nonexistent, and during the entire 2,300-year recorded history of the Hunza only two hermaphrodites are known to have been born.

On the Japanese island of Okinawa, a government census in 2001 found 457 people aged one hundred or more, or about thirty-five centenarians for every one hundred thousand islanders, the highest ratio in the world. By contrast, the United States reports about ten centenarians living for every one hundred thousand people. Equally important to longevity is the quality of life, and Okinawans are known to have the longest disability-free life expectancy of any people.

A proverb carved into a stone marker on an Okinawa beach reads: "At seventy you are but a child, at eighty you are merely a youth, and at ninety if the ancestors invite you into heaven, ask them to wait until you are one hundred and then you might consider it." That attitude gives an insight into their lifestyle, which involves a healthy diet, little or no exposure to chemical toxins, regular exercise, and a positive outlook on life. Their health-care system integrates Western and Eastern healing methods and traditions.

Rates of heart disease and cancer among Okinawans are less than one-quarter the rate in the United States. Bradley Willcox of the Harvard Medical School faculty has studied these people for over a decade and found strong evidence that their longevity and good health have little to do with their genes. Younger Okinawans who patronize fast-food restaurants located around American military bases have Japan's highest rates of obesity, heart disease, and premature death. Similarly, those Okinawans who emigrate to the United States or Brazil and adopt new eating habits lose their health and life-expectancy advantages.

Other pockets of health and longevity can be found on the island of Sardinia, among Nova Scotians in Canada, and in some Andean villages of southern Ecuador. Medical studies of centenarians in Nova Scotia revealed that half had avoided any serious or chronic illnesses. They live by the adage, "It's not true that the older you get, the sicker you become. It's the older you get, the healthier you have been."

New York University professor of nutrition Marion Nestle notes that the longest-lived populations in the world "traditionally eat diets that are largely plant-based. Such diets tend to be relatively low in calories but high in vitamins, minerals, fiber, and other components of plants [phytochemicals] that—acting together—protect against disease."

Back in 2000 the World Health Organization released the results of its measurement of each nation's life expectancy using a measurement called disability-adjusted life expectancy, in which the years of ill health are weighted according to severity and subtracted from the expected overall life expectancy to give the equivalent years of healthy life. Japan led the world among the 191 countries evaluated. The United States rated twenty-fourth under this system. Remarked Christopher Murray, director of WHO's Global Program on Evidence for Health Policy: "The position of the United States is one of the major surprises of the new rating system. Basically, you die earlier and spend more time disabled if you're an American rather than a member of most other advanced countries."

NATURE IS OUR BEST PHARMACY

Learning from nature means imitating more than just its form, as in the pharmaceutical fixation with synthesizing molecules. It means adopting the processes of nature based on our observations and experiences of nature's demonstrated healing wisdom.

"It is essential to note that nature can contribute far more to healing than new wonder drugs," says Mark J. Plotkin, the ethnobotanist. "As our culture races to embrace technology, it may seem quaint or quixotic to seek new therapeutic compounds from the world around us. Yet the history of Western civilization can be written in terms of its reliance on and utilization of natural products."

Consider what we know about those food elements from nature that constitute the "Mediterranean diet." Medical science tells us that heart patients who go on this diet reduce their risk of future heart attack and other cardiac death by up to 70 percent. By contrast, cholesterol-lowering drugs cost U.S. heart patients nearly $14 billion a year but lower their risk of recurrent heart problems by only 35 percent as much as the Mediterranean diet's combination of plants.

A milled rice fermented with red yeast, which has been used as an herbal health remedy for two thousand years in eastern Asia, has also been found effective in lowering cholesterol levels in the blood. Sold as a product called Cholestin, it contains nine compounds that work synergistically. It is as effective as many drugs prescribed for cholesterol reduction, but with fewer side effects and at less cost. "Researchers have confirmed that Cholestin reduces blood cholesterol levels by about 10 percent," reports New York University professor of nutrition Marion Nestle, and it is "priced well below its prescription counterpart." A month's supply of this natural cholesterol fighter cost Nestle about $27, compared with the $300 and up per month that the prescription anticholesterol drug Lovastatin costs consumers.

Likewise, when it comes to natural versus synthetic anti-inflammatories, the natural is proving superior in both effectiveness and cost. A professor of medicine and neurology at the University of California at Los Angeles, Greg Cole, has been studying an anti-inflammatory compound found in food called curcumin, a yellow pigment in turmeric, the curry spice used for thousands of years. Cole considers curcumin to be a far safer COX-2 inhibitor than Vioxx or similar anti-pain medications. While drugs usually block a single target molecule and reduce its activity dramatically, Cole told *Newsweek* magazine in 2005, natural anti-inflammatories gently tweak a broader range of inflammatory compounds. Needless to say, these natural-synergy healing compounds in food cost a fraction of what the pharmaceutical companies charge for their drugs.

Natural alternatives can also be found for the commonly prescribed drugs Premarin and Prempro, used by women needing hormone therapy for menopause. Jay S. Cohen, professor of medicine at the University of California at San Diego, makes a case in his book *Over Dose* for the scientifically proven benefits of natural hormones derived from vegetables. "I know several women who had miserable times with drug company hormones, yet have done very well with natural hormones," writes Cohen.

He cites four medical studies that support his natural-is-better contention. Here they are, by date of publication:

- 1989: A study in the journal *Obstetrics and Gynecology*, in which the study authors demonstrate how natural progesterone taken orally "can produce excellent blood levels without the unwanted effects (such as fluid retention, breast tenderness, weight gain and depression) of the synthetics."

- 1995: A study in the journal *Infertility and Reproductive Medicine Clinics of North America*, in which scientists tout a "natural regimen" for its "little breakthrough bleeding" compared to synthetics.
- 1997: A study in the journal *International Journal of Fertility and Women's Medicine*, in which the study authors reveal having found that "naturally occurring estrogens lower blood pressure, or have no effect on blood pressure," while synthetic estrogens and progestins elevate blood pressure.
- 1999: In the journal *Fertility and Sterility*, the study authors conclude, "In addition to the decreased potential for adverse effects [with natural hormones], there are clear advantages in convenience, cost, compliance, and quality of life."

For thirty years James A. Duke was a botanist for the United States Department of Agriculture and chief of the USDA Medicinal Plant Laboratory. He ranks as one of the world's leading authorities on botanical medicine, a term that describes medicinal trees and shrubs along with the herbs and medicinal plants used by traditional societies. "I've personally seen medicinal herbs successfully treat conditions that high-tech pharmaceuticals could not touch," declares Duke. "I've also used many of these medicinal remedies myself."

In Duke's experience the botanical remedies are often more effective, more economical, and much safer than the pharmaceuticals that try to imitate them. His extraordinary book, *The Green Pharmacy*, published in 1997, gives hundreds of natural botanical remedies for arthritis, diabetes, backache, toothache, emphysema, cataracts, menopause, and on and on. He declares his life's ambition to be "getting the FDA to make the drug companies test their new synthetic drugs not only against an inactive substance [a placebo] but also against any known or suspected herbal alternative.

"I wrote this book to show that traditional medicine has legitimate scientific value. Scientific critics counter that 'old folk tales' are no match for

Western-style scientific experimentation. But the basis of science is careful observation, and that's what traditional peoples have been doing since time immemorial—observing and experimenting with the world around them. In general, traditional people have managed to select the good medicines and have rejected the bad. Most of these folk medicines have thousands of years of experimental selection behind them, and few are associated with adverse reactions. That's something that you really can't say about our modern pharmaceuticals. All too often, synthetic drugs turn out to be hazardous."

What Duke's work signifies is the idea that our health is naturally occurring if only we will support it using the principles of nature. But with few exceptions during my own life, everyone I have ever known seems to have acted out some play on the fear that good health isn't something we have naturally acquired. Some people believe we are held captive by our genes. Others are resigned to the attitude that life should be a constant struggle against illness and disease. For most people, the convenient solution to these fears is blind obedience to physicians who compulsively prescribe synthetic chemicals. In the next chapter you will meet people who courageously broke free from that prison of mind.

CHAPTER EIGHT

WHEN WESTERN MEDICINE FAILS

"The doctor of the future will give no medicine, but will interest his patients in the care of the human frame, in diet, and in the cause and prevention of disease."

—Thomas Edison

To seventy-one-year-old Laura Baker, her doctor's words sounded like a death sentence. "You have severe emphysema," the pulmonary specialist informed her. Baker knew emphysema is a serious lung disease that makes it increasingly difficult to breathe. But the doctor added an additional distressing verdict. She would need to take steroid drugs, which have serious side effects, for the rest of her life.

She had no other options short of lung replacement surgery, said the physician, yet the toxic drugs she must now take would address only the symptoms. "Emphysema has no cure," he explained. To him that meant she could expect a restricted life connected to an oxygen tank until, after prolonged and intense pain, she died of the disease.

Though Baker left her doctor's office in Maryland in a state of shock, it only took a few days for for this former National Institute of Standards and Technology employee to make a decision that she could not—and would not—accept the fate her physician had foreseen. "Not accepting something is different from being in denial," Laura would later tell me.

After scouring books and the Internet for information about the disease, she discovered some promising alternative healing strategies. One involved exercise to strengthen her lungs. But when she told her lung specialist that she intended to join a health spa and gym, he discouraged her. "In your condition," he scolded, "you can't stay on a treadmill for more than a minute."

"Well," replied Baker, "I can at least try."

Though she gasped for air as if a pillow was pressed to her face, Laura began a stationary bike routine every day, and after a few weeks, she had increased her exercise time from five to twenty minutes. Emboldened by this progress, she contacted Angelo Druda, a practitioner of traditional Chinese herbal medicine. Laura had read how these ancient remedies might offer hope in cases where Western medicine presented only discouragement and resignation.

Druda quizzed Laura about her symptoms and medical history. He also considered the condition of her tongue—its coloration, shape, and markings—since in Chinese herbal medicine the condition of the tongue is considered a sign of problems elsewhere in the body. Druda decided that the immediate need was to enhance Laura's own regenerative capacities.

As Druda explained to me, "In the worst cases of emphysema, the air sacs in the lungs are destroyed, which is irreversible, so there would be nothing I could do to regenerate them. But the term emphysema is often applied when the air sac walls are severely damaged but not actually destroyed. Western doctors tend to apply that label too quickly. In Baker's case, I knew the recovery process had already begun, as evidenced by her gym workouts. So I devised a formula to bolster her body's restorative power by addressing her particular imbalances and deficiencies."

The liquid herbal formula Druda created consisted of fourteen herbs mixed together, including astragalus (an immune system booster), a strong ginseng extract as an energy booster for her spleen, aster to clear phlegm in her lungs, and anemarrhena to reduce her lung inflammation. The herbs would create an immune-boosting synergy within her body, an effect that is the foundation of Chinese herbal medicine.

Baker took the mixture twice a day along with a tablet containing another herb that is used for patients with respiratory problems. Within a week, Laura noticed a huge improvement in her energy and her lung stamina. As the weeks passed she kept feeling better. A true measure of her progress came during the 2002 winter holidays, at her family's annual Christmas dinner. In previous years Laura was too weak to help prepare the meal. She was unable to even carry dishes from the kitchen to the dining room. This time she felt transformed. "I was up and helping everyone," Laura recalls. "I felt full of energy. I even did some of the cooking. I carried the dishes. I helped clean up. I was ecstatic. It's so gratifying to be back in the flow of life."

Laura's account was one of several that I investigated for articles in the magazine *Alternative Medicine*, which specializes in the stories of people forced to find their own path to healing when modern Western medicine fails to find a cure. Another person I interviewed was Quinn Daly, who told me how she had overcome an illness her doctors thought was incurable.

At the age of twenty-eight, Quinn had awakened one morning at her home in San Francisco and felt an intense sensation of vertigo. The room around her whirled as if she were trapped on a carnival ride. She had lost all sense of balance. She called a 911 operator, and emergency medical technicians were dispatched. They decided she had an inner ear infection and gave her Sudafed for the infection and another drug for the dizziness. She took both drugs and promptly threw up. She passed out and was taken to a hospital, where a physician prescribed Valium and a seasickness medication.

Over the next three weeks her symptoms got worse. When the Valium would wear off the vertigo would return, and along with it an incapacitating nausea. She could no longer drive a car, exercise, go to work, or even focus on a computer screen. She had trouble keeping food down.

Quinn's mother took her to an ear, nose, and throat specialist who put her through a battery of tests. His diagnosis shocked Quinn to tears. "You have a severe form of inner ear disorder," said the specialist, "and no medication can cure it, and no surgery can fix it. You will just have to live with it."

For someone as energetic and active as she had been all of her life, this doctor's statement was a mortal wound to her spirit. During a visit from her parents and her brother, she felt gripped by despair. "We were walking down the street and I had to go very slowly, one step at a time," she related. "I moved like an old person, and that scared the heck out of my family. I had also lost fifteen pounds. They were shocked at how fragile and desperate I had become."

By happenstance she encountered a family friend, a chiropractor visiting from Los Angeles, who made an observation that provided her with hope for the first time in months. He had heard of similar symptoms in people who had an upper back problem that remained undiagnosed by conventional Western medical practitioners. He recommended that she try a bodywork technique called Rolfing.

A Rolfer in San Francisco, Marc Weill, examined her with a thermal imaging camera and found that her neck was inflamed, a condition that had probably developed over time. Eventually the inflammation caused the muscles between her shoulder blades to constrict, compressing nerves in her neck and affecting her balance. Poor nutrition had also contributed to her condition. It had absolutely nothing to do with an inner ear infection, said Weill, and it was treatable.

Blood tests enabled Weill to assess her chemistry and prescribe mineral supplements to reduce the swelling, repair the tissue damage, and boost her immune system. Immediately after her first Rolfing session she was amazed to find that the vertigo and nausea had disappeared. Two days later she had a second session and left Weill's office feeling symptom-free for good. "I walked down the street and realized that I felt normal again. I cried the whole way home."

By the time I met Quinn, four years had passed and she continued to be free of symptoms. She takes a variety of mineral supplements every day and feels stronger and healthier than ever before in her life. Quinn's story along with Laura Baker's provided me with more firsthand evidence that Western medicine's fixation on pharmaceutical drugs often does a disservice to the principles of healing. If both women had listened only to their physicians or had been reluctant to try an alternative medical approach to treatment, both would still be dependent on drugs and living without hope or a cure.

Cancer is the one diagnosis that most people seem to fear the most, and with good reason—the standard treatments of radiation and chemotherapy sometimes look and feel more damaging than the disease being treated. In a remarkable story written by a Massachusetts TV host, Portland Helmich, for *Alternative Medicine*, a woman's triumph over cancer became a testament to the ancient wisdom that food really is medicine.

A terminal case of stage IV lung cancer was the diagnosis for forty-five-year-old Janet Vitt, a registered nurse in Ohio. She had three tumors in her left lung, seven in her right, three more in her liver, and two in her pancreas and abdomen. Oncologists gave her from six weeks to six months to live. Her experimental chemotherapy resulted in a loss of forty-six pounds, and she feared these treatments would kill her faster than the cancer.

A Cleveland internist, Dennis Grossman, suggested that she try a macrobiotic diet. He had studied macrobiotics, and though most of his colleagues thought it was highly unorthodox, he felt that such a specialized diet might boost her immune system and enhance the quality of her life.

A macrobiotic food regimen, based on principles that are thousands of years old, emphasizes vegetables, fresh fruits, and whole grains but severely restricts meat, dairy products, and processed foods of any sort. The theory behind the diet is to limit the absorption of toxins while flooding the body with essential nutrients, and combining that with exercise and periods of rest and meditative solitude. It is all about creating a balanced condition in life and a natural healing synergy.

"I would have done anything at that point to live," Vitt recalls. She weighed only seventy-two pounds. "I was on oxygen. I was bald, my nails were blue, and my color was gray."

With cooking help from friends and her ex-husband, she started the macrobiotic diet and within a week had dispensed with her painkillers and anti-anxiety drugs. "I decided if I wanted to clean out my body, I couldn't be putting drugs into it." A massage therapist came three times a week to help her manage the pain. As the months passed the detox regimen improved the quality of her life, as her internist had hoped, and she no longer needed an oxygen tank.

Ten months after she began the macrobiotic diet, Vitt had another CAT scan. To the amazement of her doctors, her tumors had disappeared. "Usually that's where stories like this end," writes Helmich. "The patient walks away, mainstream docs scratch their heads in wonder and disbelief, and life goes on. But this one is different."

A George Washington University Medical Center clinical professor of urology, George Yu, presented Vitt's case and five similar cases involving the healing powers of macrobiotic diets to a panel of fifteen scientists and physicians composing the Cancer Advisory Panel for Complementary and Alternative Medicine, a branch of the National Institutes of Health in suburban Washington, D.C. In 2002 the panel unanimously recommended federal government funding for a clinical study on the impact of macrobiotics on cancer.

As for why the diet apparently works with some cancer patients, Yu speculates that the reliance on fermented foods like miso generates a bacteria that produces enzymes, and these enzymes help to eliminate toxins and keep the body in balance. He estimates that one-third of people with serious illnesses who go on long-term macrobiotic diets recover within six months. Janet Vitt's recovery has lasted more than ten years without a recurrence of cancers, and the diet also freed her from migraine headaches and joint pain.

No single treatment modality has the right to claim a monopoly on the truth about the cures for illness and disease. We each must find our own path to health that works uniquely for us. Lynne McTaggart's experience provides another textbook example. She had been ill for three years in the 1980s and no one could determine why. She had chronic candidiasis (a vaginal yeast infection) caused by a weakened immune system, but none of her physicians or the specialists they recommended could diagnose this cause from her symptoms. Eventually she realized that "if I was going to get better, I was going to have to take charge of the entire process myself—from diagnosis to, possibly, even the cure."

She succeeded at healing herself using vitamin and mineral supplements and a restrictive diet. Having experienced firsthand that people can get well without drugs and surgery, she wrote a book, *What Doctors Don't Tell You,* and became a campaigner for patients taking personal responsibility for their own care. "Healing isn't simply a matter of finding the right drug or right operation, but a complex process of accepting responsibility for your own life."

For many people who grew up awed by and dependent on technology and the laboratory drugs of Western medicine, breaking free of that paradigm, or even considering the use of strange-sounding treatments from other cultures, requires a leap of faith. To make that leap more inviting, some myths need shattering.

MYTHS WE CHERISH

ANCIENT PHYSICIANS WERE UNSOPHISTICATED

If you had lived in Egypt about 1900 BC and suffered a work accident or a war wound, you probably would have been diagnosed and treated by physicians who had been trained from a medical text found on a papyrus—its eleven hieroglyphic panels spanning fifteen feet when unrolled—that contained instructions for treating forty-eight types of injuries to the human body.

This ancient medical text still exists and was the centerpiece of an exhibit, "The Art of Medicine in Ancient Egypt," at New York City's Metropolitan Museum of Art in late 2005, sponsored by the New York Academy of Medicine. It was an opportunity for Western practitioners of medicine to gain an appreciation for a tradition most had previously ignored or disparaged. "When you see these things, you really have to marvel at the ingenuity of these people," commented David Mininberg, a New York City physician who acted as a consultant to the exhibit. "They were meticulous recorders of what they observed."

Many of these doctors four thousand years ago were specialists in gynecological, dental, or other health areas. The medical texts from this period in history clearly reflect how these healers understood the limitations of their powers and their knowledge. When they were treating work accident injuries or war wounds, for instance, they made a diagnosis and then initiated treatment based on three categories of care detailed on the papyrus: an ailment I will handle, an ailment I will fight with, or an ailment for which nothing is done.

"In light of today's practices, in my opinion, it's an incredibly enlightened view," Dr. Mininberg told a reporter for *HealthDay*, describing the three treatment categories. "In other words, in the first case he says, 'I know what this is, I can treat it, and I'm expecting a good outcome.' In the second category, he hedges his bets a little bit. And the third category is what I think is most impressive: not to treat. . . . rather than undertake end-of-life, heroic measures with no chance of success, he simply gives supportive care."

Doctors in ancient Egypt typically used honey on wounds and burns to assist in healing, though they apparently had no idea it was harmful bacteria they were destroying. Observes ethnobotanist Mark J. Plotkin: "A spate of recent publications has highlighted the successful use of honey to treat infected wounds and burns that do not respond well to conventional treatment." Other Egyptian medical texts from the period of 166 BC have been found advising that spoiled barley bread, which had a medicinal effect similar to penicillin, be pressed onto infected wounds.

Through trial and error and intuition the ancient Egyptian healers discovered what works and continued using those remedies for two thousand years. They employed pomegranate as an effective astringent, used lotus root for its morphinelike analgesics, and they knew how to suture and cauterize. Their technology and their knowledge of disease and anatomy may have been limited, but their wisdom about how to use plants for healing was far advanced. They even knew how to wield the power of the placebo effect to heal when nothing else worked, by calling upon spells and magic potions dedicated to a deity, Sekmet, in whose powers many Egyptians had a fervent respect and belief.

In ancient Mesopotamia around 2000 BC, Assyrian and Babylonian medicine had also reached a surprisingly high level of sophistication. Two Illinois university academics, JoAnn Scurlock, a professor of ancient history, and Burton Andersen, a professor of medicine, studied the medical texts surviving from that period in the original cuneiform, the first known system of writing. They produced a nine-hundred-page book, *Diagnoses in Assyrian and Babylonian Medicine,* which concluded that people living four thousand years ago received medical treatment far superior to what

Americans got when George Washington was alive in the eighteenth century.

Among the dozens of revelations in their 2005 book:

- Ancient physicians were trained as specialists in dentistry, neurology, gynecology, pediatrics, and other areas of medicine, and they utilized the medicinal properties of more than three hundred Mesopotamian plants in their treatments.
- Careful observation and experimentation produced treatments that evolved over hundreds of years. Some of these ancient treatments are still in common use today within Western medicine, one being the practice of surgically draining fluid from between the lungs and chest of pneumonia patients by making an opening in the fourth rib and inserting a drainage tube.
- These ancient doctors were able to measure pulse rates and used metal hammers to tap below the knee to test reflexes, just as we do today.
- They cleaned surgical wounds using bandages treated with ginger and cedar, both antiseptics; they treated night blindness with raw liver, which we now know corrects the vitamin A deficiencies that cause night blindness; they used marijuana to treat pain and nausea, just as we do for cancer patients today; they treated women with irregular monthly cycles using a medicine made from date pits, which we now know contains estrogens.

Herbal medicine also reached a high stage of development among some European tribes who were contemporaries of the Egyptians and Babylonians. You may recall how in 1991 the frozen body of a 5,300-year-old man was discovered high in the Alps, on the border of present-day Italy and Austria. He carried with him three wood conk mushrooms tethered to his right side along with a fragment of birch polypore. These herbs have strong immune-system-boosting and antibiotic properties and are effective against various strains of E. coli bacteria. Wanderers or shepherds like the iceman, as he has come to be known, commonly carried medicine pouches and self-administered the herbs as needed based on instructions from the tribe's herbal shaman.

In the Bible's New Testament we have more evidence for this ancient healing knowledge. "The Gift of the Magi (gold, frankincense, and myrrh) given to Jesus, Joseph, and Mary two thousand years ago was not merely two room deodorizers to make the barn smell better," observes Mark J. Plotkin, the ethnobotanist and author of *Medicine Quest.* "It was the gift of life itself—the most essential medicine of the ancient world."

Myrrh is a tree resin and was prized as an antibiotic and used by physician healers in Persia, Egypt, Greece, and Rome to clean and dress wounds. Frankincense is another resin with similar qualities. Modern experiments have found both to be anti-inflammatories and antifungals, and myrrh has pain-relief powers as well, which, as Plotkin points out, "is probably why it was administered to Jesus prior to his crucifixion."

MYTHS WE CHERISH

ANCIENT REMEDIES ARE UNSCIENTIFIC

For centuries tribal peoples in Central America, Burma, Australia, and elsewhere used maggots and leeches for healing in their traditional medical practices. During most of the twentieth century Western medical "experts" ridiculed this use of flesh-eating maggots and bloodsucking leeches as examples of primitive barbarism and superstitious ignorance.

These tools of ancient wisdom have finally been rediscovered by medical science because their high-tech treatments for wounds sometimes fail in cases where maggots and leeches succeed. The turnaround in Western medicine's attitudes began in the early 1990s as a result of studies conducted by Ronald Sherman, who raised maggots in his laboratory at the University of California at Irvine and tested them on hard-to-treat infected wounds.

Maggots not only eat dead flesh while ignoring living tissue, they secrete chemical substances that destroy bacteria and stimulate the growth of healthy tissue. While they do inspire some understandable squeamishness on the part of humans, they are incredibly effective and cheap tools for healing. Diabetics who develop foot ulcers, for instance, might spend thousands of dollars on high-tech treatments and surgeries that fail, compared with a pittance spent on a few maggots that save the foot from amputation.

Medical studies have found maggots to be twice as effective as modern medicine at cleansing dead tissue from wounds, and patients treated with maggots spend many fewer days taking antibiotics and other drugs. At the University of Miami Cedars Wound Center, where maggots are now routinely used, the director Robert Kirsner calls them an indispensable tool because "maggots do work very well."

Leeches play a similarly new but important role in modern medicine by healing hard-to-treat cases of surgically reattached or transplanted body parts. They drain excess blood from surgical areas and naturally inject patients with a healing chemical cocktail that includes an anesthetic, an antibiotic, an anticoagulant, and a substance that is effective at dilating blood vessels to enhance blood flow. Microsurgeons say that leeches have become their most important secret weapon in restoring blood circulation and insuring the success of problematic surgeries.

During 2005 both maggots and leeches became the first living organisms to receive FDA regulatory blessings as "medical devices." An FDA official described for *The New York Times* his agency's logic in defining these critters as mechanical devices: "The primary mode of action for maggots is chewing. For leeches, it's the eating of blood. Those are mechanical processes."

Here are just a few of the other ways in which modern medicine is rediscovering and using ancient medical wisdom:

- An Asian species of fungus called *Cordyceps*, used by the ancient Chinese for impotence, has been shown in recent clinical trials to be effective for treating loss of sexual desire among the elderly.
- An ancient treatment for arthritis among Amazon tribes is ant venom, which contains a previously unknown complex sugar molecule that has been shown in laboratory experiments to be effective against pain and inflammation.

- The ancient Greeks and Romans used the wild fennel plant as a female contraceptive, and modern studies with lab animals have confirmed that it is effective in stopping reproduction.

Both traditional Chinese medicine and ayurvedic medicine from India are ancient systems that take into acccount specific times of the day to treat specific ailments or parts of the body. Western medicine had discounted these ideas—until recently. What changed Western attitudes was the discovery that the human body's biological clock alters biochemistry according to phases of the sleep cycle and other factors of time and day. Using those rhythms can enhance a treatment's effectiveness. Asthma is a prime example. Under the ancient systems an energy imbalance in the lungs was said to manifest between three a.m. and five a.m.; clinical research has found that, yes indeed, during that time frame changing levels of cortical hormones and epinephrine in asthma sufferers make it more difficult to keep their airways open. Similar patterns have been confirmed for arthritis and other ailments.

At London's Kew Gardens' Jodrell Laboratory a group of scientists began a series of molecular tests and clinical trials during the summer of 2005, examining the herbal cures described in a famous text called *Herbal*, written in 1628 but based on hundreds of years of folk-healing wisdom preceding the seventeenth century. The first plant they analyzed was figwort, identified in the ancient text as containing a substance that "dissolves clotted and congealed blood within the body," and was traditionally used to heal wounds. The scientists discovered that figwort did indeed initiate a healing process in cell cultures they subjected to analysis.

Next they looked at sage, an herb that has been connected with wisdom down through the ages, and in collaboration with researchers at King's College London, found that sage does affect receptors in the brain. People who took sage oil showed a marked improvement in their memory. Amazed by the effectiveness of the first two herbal remedies they examined, they expanded their study scope and mandate to use molecular technology in attempts to unlock the potential healing secrets of all 1,600 plants native to Britain. "It's a question of old traditional knowledge and new technology coming together and giving us new answers," Monique

Simmonds, chief plant scientist at Kew Gardens, explained to the *London Observer*.

Similarly methodical examinations of plants native to North America might yield many more healing surprises. Most of the hundreds of Native American tribal traditions maintain some verbal or written inventory of plants with known healing qualities. Cherokee medicine, for example, with its theme of mixing medicine from nature's gifts, uses dozens of herbs with established health benefits. Alfalfa, which is rich in six vitamins and calcium, has been a traditional immune system booster. Marigold flowers have been a longtime cure-all because of their antimicrobial, antifungal, and antibacterial properties.

Nature provides the most ancient wisdom of all about how to heal the human body, and we have barely begun to tap its resources. Some revealing statistics about the rich diversity of its potential for health and healing can be found in a collection of essays on ecology, *Nature's Services*.

In tropical forests an estimated 125,000 flowering plants exist, few of which have been studied by laboratories for their medicinal properties. Given that many species have five separate components with medicinal potential—fruit, flowers, leaves, stems, and roots—up to 750,000 potential healing extracts might be found. Not only that, but our planet supports about 75,000 plants that are edible, yet only three thousand or so plant species have ever been utilized as food during human history. Of that number maybe 150 have been cultivated on a large scale. The unexplored wealth of food nutrients and healing compounds from botanicals—edible or not—is amazingly diverse and immense, a true Garden of Eden.

An executive with the Bristol-Myers Squibb pharmaceutical company made this frank admission to a *Newsweek* reporter in 2005: "The complexity and diversity of natural products can't be matched by even the most innovative human scientist. I think we're going to see a resurgence of interest in natural products."

Though this interest only seems to involve using natural products as templates to create synthetic drugs that can be patented, it still represents a rare confession by a pharmaceutical company about how designing drugs from scratch has failed to achieve the promises made to us of a healthier life through chemistry.

REDISCOVERING ANCIENT WISDOM TRADITIONS

"The medical paradigm that currently prevails in our U.S. society and which the AMA [American Medical Association] stalwartly represents," wrote John Robbins in his book *Reclaiming Our Health*, "has become so deeply entrenched that we often do not realize that it is simply one option among many. But there are other forms of medicine that represent different ways of understanding life and of promoting healing, and that, contrary to what the dominant medical establishment would have us believe, have demonstrated outstanding records of success."

Traditional systems of medicine from India and China have both developed over four thousand years of knowledge based on trial-and-error testing of untold millions of people in the longest and most widespread clinical trial tests of plant-based healing in human history. Both systems place more emphasis on illness and disease prevention—especially using food and diet—than does Western-based (allopathic) medicine, which tends to view preventive measures only in terms of public sanitation and public immunizations. Neither of these traditional systems believe it's appropriate or effective to isolate specific compounds or to synthesize molecules from a medicinal plant.

To explore the differences between these two major ancient wisdom traditions and the modern Western system of medicine, I enlisted two friends who are experts in their fields to discuss the relative strengths and weaknesses of all three systems of healing. For twenty-five years Scott Treadway has taught, lectured, and published in the field of nutritional science, with a specialty in ayurvedic medicine, the ancient healing tradition of India. Angelo Druda is a member of the Australian Natural Therapists Association and has been a certified practitioner of traditional Chinese medicine for more than a decade.

They identify three principles in particular that both traditions have in common and that sets them apart from synthetic drug approaches to health.

Traditional Systems Use Food as Medicine: What we eat, the fuel we burn to power our body and mind, can be used in prevention and to heal and regenerate, or else—if consumed mindlessly—it will toxify the body and mind, weaken the immune system, and invite illness and disease. That principle guides both ancient healing systems. Everything begins with food.

"One of the first things we do in treatment is address the food body and the imbalances created by diet," says Angelo. Advice about basic lifestyle and dietary changes comes with every diagnosis and every regimen of herbal treatments, which is a synergistic approach that's designed to enable anyone to detoxify and regain an overall health balance. By eliminating toxins from food and chemical toxins from the body through detoxification, the body's own regenerative chemistry is magnified and the immune system is strengthened.

Traditional Medicine Is Synergistic: Modern allopathic medicine focuses on chemical magic bullets; the treatment of symptoms, and the mechanics of the human body, while the two ancient traditions believe health is naturally occurring and responds to synergistic laws of nature. "Traditional medicine allows 'nature' in the form of our immune system to do much of the healing," Scott observes. That means using combinations of healing herbs to empower the immune system to regenerate the body. By refusing to tamper with plant chemistry these two ancient systems respect and preserve the synergies that activate healing and health.

"Traditional systems are rational systems, which observe the interrelatedness of the body's organs," adds Angelo. "We look for synergies right from the start in prevention and treatment, whereas the empirical system of allopathic medicine never even thinks in those terms." In that sense practitioners of ayurvedic and Chinese medicine are like detectives treating each person as a unique individual, based on discovering what can jump-start the patient's own regenerative chemistry.

Traditional Medicine Is Integrative: If you need emergency care for an injury or an illness, or if you have a heart attack or a stroke, both Scott and Angelo would urge you to immediately seek allopathic treatment because modern Western medicine offers superb emergency service. By integrating this reactive emergency medicine with the preventive and synergistic approaches of traditional systems, consumers of medical care have the opportunity to experience the extraordinary benefits of both perspectives on health and healing. China and India are each in the forefront of combining naturopathic and allopathic principles and practices into a strong and visionary twenty-first-century integrated medicine.

CHAPTER NINE

BRINGING IT ALL HOME

"From the right to know and the duty to inquire flows the obligation to act."

—Sandra Steingraber in *Living Downstream: An Ecologist Looks at Cancer and the Environment*

If we ignore ancient wisdom and fail to embrace naturally occurring foods and medicines, we will face unpalatable risk trade-offs across an increasingly broad range of choices in our everyday lives. Already we find ourselves asking should we consume margarine and its trans-fat toxins, or do we instead eat butter and absorb the toxic chemical residues "offloaded" by milk cows? Do we give our children infant formula containing potentially harmful synthetic chemicals, or do we feed them breast milk contaminated with their mother's own chemical body load? Should we eat fish for the polyunsaturated fatty acids they contain that help protect us against stroke and heart disease, or should we avoid eating fish entirely because they are contaminated with methyl mercury that impairs human IQ and cognitive development?

Because we all live in the same chemical neighborhood, which is to say, planet Earth, we all have been participants in this huge chemical experiment that we call modern civilization. As a consequence, we can expect our risk trade-off quandaries to multiply and sharpen with time because the chemical onslaught against our health is quickening and deepening. Flame retardants in plastics, known as PBDEs, illustrate one facet of the problem. Measurements conducted by the U.S. Centers for Disease Control and Prevention indicate that PBDE levels in our bodies *are doubling every eighteen months.*

Synthetic-chemical production levels overall have been doubling every decade since the 1940s. At least five new synthetic chemicals are developed for commercial use every single day, yet no one has any realistic idea how harmful these chemicals are to us, either alone or acting in synergy with other chemicals. Our ignorance on these matters long ago surpassed our wisdom. Even global warming, to the extent that it's caused or exacerbated by human actions, mostly stems from the release of synthetic chemical toxins.

Since the start of the Hundred-Year Lie in 1906, the year the U.S. Congress enacted the Pure Food and Drug Act, we have a century of false and misleading guarantees from which to draw lessons. Here are the ones I draw from the research contained in this book and the patterns that emerged as a consequence of one hundred years of mythmaking.

- We can inherit harm. Toxic synthetic chemicals can negatively alter our DNA to program us and our descendants to experience illness and disease.
- Synthetic chemicals take advantage of nutrient-poor diets to damage our immune systems, which facilitates the onset of illness and disease.
- Some synthetic chemicals interact with each other to produce toxic synergies that activate our genetic predisposition to illness and disease.
- Synthetic chemicals can create toxic synergies to trigger the development of "new" illnesses and diseases, such as chronic fatigue syndrome and Gulf War syndrome.
- Drugs being prescribed for the illnesses and diseases caused by synthetic chemicals are introducing more toxins into the body, further confusing and compromising our immune systems.
- Human bodies weren't designed to absorb synthetic chemicals,

even at low doses, throughout a lifetime, without harm being inflicted.

• Our best hope for health and longevity is to embrace naturally occurring synergies found in the foods and medicines of nature. Our rediscovery of ancient wisdom can rescue us from the follies of this failed experiment with our biochemical nature.

Try and imagine what will happen if, for the rest of the twenty-first century, the synthetics belief system of the previous hundred years remains supported by our bodies and our bank accounts. We can already see the signs of an accelerated degeneration of our species. It has spread across multiple layers of life and throughout nature. It's characterized by infertility, reproductive abnormalities, birth defects, weakened immune systems, and a contagion of illness and disease that threatens to bankrupt every industrialized society with runaway medical costs.

This isn't hyperbole or fearmongering. Our nation really is going broke from medical costs that consume nearly two trillion dollars in annual spending—and most other industrialized nations are not far behind us. Every thirty seconds in the United States, someone must file personal bankruptcy in the aftermath of a serious health problem. Premiums for employee-sponsored health insurance have been rising five times faster on average than workers' earnings since the year 2000. Many companies are dropping or trimming their employee health coverage. An estimated forty-five million Americans are now uninsured because they cannot afford to pay private insurance premiums. This in turn puts a huge strain on federal and state government insurance programs. That bedrock of American health care, the government program for the elderly called Medicare, will go broke by 2019, warns Comptroller General David Walker, who heads the Government Accountability Office. "The Medicare problem is about seven times greater than the Social Security problem," Walker told members of the U.S. Congress in 2005. "It is much bigger, it is much more immediate, and it is going to be much more difficult to effectively address."

It's as if we're witnessing one of those slow-motion train wrecks in which three tracks are converging. On track one roars the runaway train of synthetic chemical production. On track two comes the runaway train of health-care costs. On track three barrels the runaway train of environmental effects that are diminishing human and animal fertility. When the wreck debris finally settles, a powerful synergy of unpredictable social forces will be unleashed.

Medical scientists rarely make alarmist statements or apocalyptic predictions in public for fear of ridicule or being ostracized by their peers. That tendency toward caution makes the joint declaration known as "The Vallombrosa Consensus Statement on Environmental Contaminants" all the more startling in its directness and import. Sounding an alarm about the link between synthetic chemicals and infertility, forty U.S. and Canadian physicians and scientists representing the National Institute of Environmental Health Sciences, Stanford University's School of Medicine, Harvard's School of Public Health, and a dozen other prominent research institutions signed and released a public statement in October 2005 affirming key findings in this book:

- 12 percent of the U.S. reproductive population now experiences infertility, and that rate is rising overall, particularly among women under twenty-five years of age.
- A "growing body of literature and research" implicates "a wide array of modern chemicals" in this infertility trend.
- Similar effects of infertility, along with desmasculinization and birth defects, are being documented among wildlife populations.
- Low levels of exposures to chemical contaminants are causing these effects in both humans and animal life.
- Current technologies to measure the health impacts of multiple chemicals in the human body "significantly underestimate effects of chemical mixtures."
- The link between synthetic chemicals and infertility "is a question of profound human, scientific and public policy significance" and the scientific evidence for such a connection "is sufficient to raise troubling questions about the future of human reproductive health."

WE ARE IN DEEP TROUBLE

The toxins genie is out of the bottle, and no amount of handwringing or belated actions by government will bring it under control again, at least not in our lifetimes. There are no modern medical instruction manuals on how to survive the toxin genie's unpredictable and harmful effects. All we know for certain is that we are swimming without life preservers in this chemical soup, and no one can say with authority what will happen to us.

For those of you who choose to believe that government or industry or science will rescue us in the near future, consider the following reasons why that hope may be naive:

1. We cannot completely rely upon government at any level to protect us. Environmental scientists have been warning us for decades that chemical companies inject so many hundreds of new synthetic chemicals into our lives each year that toxicologists and regulatory agencies of government can no longer even develop new tests to detect their presence. Any attempt to develop adequate tests to identify toxic synergies among the one hundred thousand or so chemicals in use would be financially and technologically akin to the Manhattan Project creating an atomic bomb. Though we have a tradition of generally trusting government and scientists and manufacturers, we have sometimes done so to our detriment. "From nuclear radiation and CFCs to the various chlorinated hydrocarbon pesticides," says Dr. Suzanne Wuerthele of the EPA, "we're always playing catch-up, finding out about health and ecological effects after it's too late."

We must learn to think for ourselves, says neurosurgeon Dr. Russell Blaylock, who chides us for having "placed too much faith in guardian federal agencies that (we) ignore obvious dangers." A study by scientists at the University of Missouri has found that the chemical-risk-assessment standards used by government agencies are in urgent need of "radical change." Standards currently used to measure the harm inflicted by synthetic chemicals "need strengthening by a factor of 10,000 or greater," the study concluded. Yet, there is no funding program within the U.S. government, nor even one being seriously proposed, to develop the necessary technology to identify low-level or synergistic chemical threats.

2. We cannot rely upon manufacturers to place our health above profit margins. The German investment rating agency Oekom Research evaluated twenty-three international chemical companies using two hundred criteria in 2005 to see how they cope with environmental and health risks. Nearly every company examined made "generally poor efforts to record and evaluate substance risks." How manufacturers have dealt with known hazards associated with the weed killer atrazine and the Teflon chemical used in food packaging provide two glaring examples of the generally low priority given public health concerns.

In 2004, *The Washington Post* reported how the Swiss manufacturer of atrazine hired a lobbying firm in Washington, D.C., and successfully thwarted attempts by the EPA to regulate the substance after science studies documented its hormone disruption in wildlife. Frogs and other animals exposed to atrazine had developed both male and female sex organs after tiny exposures, just 0.1 parts per billion, or the equivalent of one drop of atrazine in 200,000 gallons of water. The European Union banned the use of atrazine in 2005, but the EPA permits its ongoing use without restrictions because, according to the agency, "the government has not settled on an officially accepted test for measuring hormone disruption."

Former DuPont Company senior engineer Glen Evers publicly revealed in 2005 that the company knew that the Teflon chemical called PFOA, widely used in fast-food packaging, microwave popcorn bags, and candy wrappers, leaches into the food in greater concentrations than had been reported to the FDA. "You don't see it, you don't feel it, you can't taste it," Evers, a twenty-two-year employee of DuPont, told reporters. "But when you open that bag and you start dipping your French fries in there, you are extracting fluorochemical and you're eating it."

First approved by the FDA for food packaging in 1967, the chemical zonyl—used to prevent grease stains from soaking through paper wrapping—breaks down into the chemical called PFOA once it enters the human body. PFOA stays in the body, bioaccumulating for extended periods, and has been linked to cancer and other health abnormalities. An internal DuPont memo from 1987 detailed how zonyl was being secreted into foods at a rate three times higher than had been predicted to occur, but this new alarming data was never reported to the FDA. Thanks to whistleblower Evers, a lawsuit filed by the U.S. government over this two-decade-long failure to reveal the health threat resulted in DuPont paying $10.2 million in fines during late 2005.

3. We cannot completely rely upon science to predict what is healthy or harmful. Medical science as an institution finds itself in a tight box as a result of its dependence on the synthetics paradigm. Nothing better illustrates the mind-set contouring that box than the U.S. government's thirty-five-year war on cancer. After throwing hundreds of billions of taxpayer dollars into research to develop synthetic drug cures for this contagion—that is really not one disease, but hundreds of cellular diseases governed by a synergy of causative factors—we find ourselves flailing around in the darkness of a blind alley.

Cancer statistics for the period 1998–2002, compiled by the National Cancer Institute, tell a story of younger and younger victims among the 2.7 million U.S. citizens who died of cancer and another 833,000 newly diagnosed cases in just those five years. Nearly half of all deaths and new cases of cancer in eight categories—trachea, bones and joints, cervix, testicles, cranial nerves, lymphatic system, thyroid and endocrine system—occurred in people less than thirty-four years of age. Some youth death figures simply stagger the imagination. For instance, nearly 64 percent of all deaths from the form of leukemia called acute lymphocytic occur in teenagers and young children.

A myth-busting *New York Times* article in December 2005 surveyed medical experts about the "crisis in cancer research" and came to a series of sobering conclusions. "Cancer has had the greatest chasm (of any disease) between hope and reality." Among cancer drugs gaining FDA approval over the last twenty years, "fewer than one in five have been shown to extend lives, life extensions usually measured in weeks or months, not years . . . Patients who take every one of the high-tech drugs has to spend, on average, $250,000, suffer serious side effects, and gain, on average, months of life."

Given this appalling record one might hope that the medical science luminaries who direct our cancer war might be open to accepting the prospect of their chemical "cures" being more of a problem than a solution. That would, of course, be asking them to reject the synthetics paradigm and to think outside of their self-created box. A second *New York Times* story, also in December 2005, further stripped away the science emperor's public relations clothing.

Medical researchers are on a quest, the article related, "looking for reliable ways to detect environmental exposures and determine whether they are linked to cancer risk. They are studying the bewildering array of factors that can determine a chemical's effects on individual people." The problem with this approach is that it must involve a study of synergies, but medical scientists, by their own admission, have only the faintest idea how to accurately gauge the impact of synergistic factors in cancer development or in the development of any other disease.

So scientists content themselves once again with chasing down blind alleys seeking a specific chemical as the cause of a specific type of cancer. But even if they were to find a specific chemical's link to cancer, confessed Dr. Aaron Blair, an epidemiologist at the National Cancer Institute, any decision to ban the chemical would be "difficult because (such decisions) were, in part, political, balancing the costs of getting rid of the chemical against the benefits." Here we have another admission that public health doesn't always take center stage with government or industry or science.

PROTECTING OURSELVES

If we cannot trust government, nor industry, nor science to protect us from chemical harm until that harm has been inflicted, who or what should we trust? The answer may simply be that we must trust ourselves.

If we are going to be guinea pigs, let it be on our own terms. We must learn how to trust our own experience, our own powers of observation, and our own intuition. Whether that level of personal accountability is embraced or not may largely depend on your vision of the human future.

In *Washington Post* reporter Joel Garreau's book *Radical Evolution*, he documents trends in genetics and technology that he predicts will totally transform life as we know it in this century. He projects the emergence of two groups of humans: the "enhanced" and the "natural." The enhanced will use synthetic chemicals in an attempt to increase memory, stamina, beauty, and life expectancy, while naturals will resist anything synthetic.

Rarely does life or a historical moment present us with a clear choice about one way of being versus another. None of us may live long enough to experience a day when we would actually be confronted by a need to choose between leading a synthetic or a natural life. But we are already making innumerable small, seemingly inconsequential decisions and steps that define who we are becoming every single day of our lives.

Our most pressing practical challenge is how best to protect ourselves and those we care about. How can we manage these multiplying risks without being stampeded by fear, or sabotaged by complacency and denial, or paralyzed by cynicism and despair?

There is a straightforward three-step process you or anyone can initiate once you become serious about protecting your health.

1. Limit your exposure to synthetic chemicals of all types at all times.
2. Get yourself tested to determine your chemical body burden.
3. Develop a detox strategy for yourself to eliminate the toxins detected in your body.

The lie we've been telling ourselves for a century—that synthetic chemicals in our food and medicine are benign—has weakened our immune systems and made us more susceptible to every infusion of new chemical toxins or pandemic of microbes that emerges to challenge our health and survival. So long as we continue supporting this broken system with our bodies and our pocketbooks, it will propel us at an accelerating speed down a slippery slope leading to the further degeneration of our species.

As a culture we are in the throes of a death process. It will either be the death of the lie, or the death of all of our conceptions of what it means to be human.

FIVE SOCIETAL CHANGES WORTH SUPPORTING

1. Pressure the Toxins Manufacturers—Under public scrutiny and pressure from San Francisco's Breast Cancer Fund and the Campaign for Safe Cosmetics in 2005, two cosmetics companies, Revlon and L'Oreal USA, agreed to purge their products of chemicals identified by the European Union as possible causes of cancer, birth defects, and infertility. Unilever followed suit with its cosmetics, and Procter & Gamble agreed to remove phthalates from its nail polish. None of these voluntary actions would have happened without public pressure from consumer groups.

2. Create a Naturally Occurring Standard—To insure that vitamin and mineral supplements are natural and taken directly from plant sources, and do not contain synthetics of any sort, a Naturally Occurring Standard needs to be implemented with an NOS certification logo. This will help to eliminate the confusion and deception we now see practiced by some elements of the supplements industry that attempt to make naturals and synthetics indistinguishable. Such a certification might also be a worthwhile addition to—or substitution for—the "organic" label on food products, a label under constant threat of dilution by food processing companies.

3. Encourage Preventive Health Care—New tools are emerging that will affirm the old adage "good health is easier to preserve than it is to repair." We know that illness and disease can be triggered by an interaction between our genes and chemical toxins we have ingested or absorbed. Self-diagnosis will soon be advanced by genomic medicine, which will enable us to decipher our genetic weaknesses and identify those specific toxins that can initiate disease processes in us. This technology can result in more individualized types of health care that will include accurate in-home testing. Another advance is the BioPhotonic Scanner. This device measures the levels of antioxidants in the human body. Invented by physicists at the University of Utah in 2001, it emits a low-

energy blue laser light into the palm of your hand and reads the health of your immune system, enabling you to identify vitamin and mineral supplements that might remedy deficiencies and strengthen your immunity. Nutrient testing should become a standard part of physical exams to measure immune system health.

4. Make Dining a Health Education Opportunity—We can hope that in restaurants of the near future, menus will describe the health benefits—not just the caloric intake—of each food choice. One page might feature dishes designed to promote a healthy heart. Another page would spotlight dishes with cancer-prevention ingredients. To make that a reality, we need to be vocal consumers and let the restaurant industry know that our patronage will be dependent on their exercise of social responsibility.

5. Accept Alternative Remedies—Surveys of allopathic (Western) medical practitioners reveal a widening acceptance of integrative healing practices and strategies. A poll of seven hundred U.S. physicians in 2005, conducted by a research institute associated with the Jewish Theological Seminary of America, found that 64 percent had recommended treatments from the field of alternative medicine to their patients. Do your own homework. Read and research the track records of alternative and integrative approaches to health and healing.

A DETOX JOURNEY

Ninety miles north of San Francisco in Lake County, where I've lived for six years, residents take some comfort and pride in having the cleanest air and purest water of any county in the state of California. We are encircled by mountain ranges, and the primary industries are tourism, hot springs resorts, Indian casinos, and vineyards. The Mendocino National Forest covers the entire northern half of the county, and Clear Lake, the largest body of water in the state, sprawls over the central portion. When I moved here there were only seven traffic lights and 65,000 residents in a geographical area the size of the state of Rhode Island.

To measure how contaminated with chemical toxins I've become despite my relatively pristine and remote surroundings, and to test whether detox strategies for removing synthetic chemicals actually work, I became a guinea pig in an experiment that I helped devise. Eight vials of blood and a urine sample were taken from me at a hospital and sent by overnight express to the Accu-Chem Laboratory in Dallas, a toxicology facility with the capability of measuring minute amounts of hundreds of synthetic chemicals in the human body.

A similar "biomonitoring" experiment was done two years earlier on five San Francisco Bay area residents whose blood was tested by the Mount Sinai School of Medicine in New York to seek traces of chemicals commonly found in consumer goods and the environment. Each test subject had an average of fifty-five chemicals in their body known to be toxic to the human reproductive system and an average of sixty-two chemicals toxic to the nervous system. This was considered to be within the "normal" levels of a body burden that we all carry.

Body burden tests have been described as a type of thermometer that gives us a reading on our body's chemical fever. My interest in being tested wasn't so much in finding out how many synthetic toxins had taken up residence in me—there were bound to be hundreds—but rather to learn which toxins had contaminated me at levels higher than the lab's average for other people. I also wanted to measure the extent to which I could reverse this process by leaching the toxins out of body tissues and blood using a natural-foods detox regimen.

Results from the initial round of testing showed numerous toxins in my blood at abnormally elevated levels. These included the pesticides DDE, HCB, and Mirex, along with arsenic, a heavy metal that could have come from drinking water or seafood. The most puzzling to me was DDE, a breakdown component of DDT, a toxic pesticide banned in the United States for the past three decades. Apparently DDE still commonly shows up in imported fruits and vegetables, and it's known to persist for years as a contaminant in soils previously sprayed with DDT. Mirex also persists in the environment even though this fire retardant and ant killer was taken out of commercial use over a decade ago.

With these body-contaminant chemicals as my target, I needed a supportive environment within which to test a detoxification strategy. A friend strongly recommended the Hippocrates Health Institute in Florida for its program designed to detoxify the body and rejuvenate the immune system.

The founder of Hippocrates, Ann Wigmore, a Lithuanian who emigrated to Boston, had been diagnosed with colon cancer and then her legs had been crushed in an auto accident during the 1950s. She instinctively began chewing on common lawn grass and credited the juice with healing both her cancer and the leg injuries. Later she settled on wheatgrass juice as the most nutritious and medicinal "living food" and that became the therapeutic centerpiece of the Hippocrates program. (The Optimum Health Institutes in San Diego and Austin also incorporate many of her ideas.)

Over the past few decades Hippocrates and its message have attracted a celebrity clientele that includes the actor Paul Newman, civil rights icon

Coretta Scott King, comedian Dick Gregory, and musicians Kenny Loggins and Mick Fleetwood. People must arrive prepared to exercise self-discipline because the regimen is strict. Nothing but raw vegetables and juices are allowed in the diet. No synthetic chemicals of any sort are allowed on the premises, so that means discarding most deodorants, hairsprays, sunscreens, and cosmetics. It's a detox strategy designed to lift the burden that synthetic chemicals in our food, medicine, and personal-care products impose on our immune systems.

"Food as Medicine" Miracles

Thanksgiving dinner at Hippocrates featured an organic vegan (no dairy products) feast of garlic artichokes, zucchini fetuccine, and mounds of raw veggies, especially sprouts, consumed by 250 or so Hippocrates patients, staff, and guests. Much to my surprise, this rather narrow selection didn't provoke the cravings for turkey and traditional trimmings that I feared might obsess me, if only because after four days of being here and eating a raw-foods diet my appetite had largely disappeared and with it, ten pounds of my excess body weight.

Hippocrates and its staff of eighty-five healers and support personnel work within forty acres of lush tropical landscaping situated on the edge of West Palm Beach. The setting with its two small lakes, four bathing pools, sauna, gym, and massage center resembles an expensive spa, or a spiritual retreat with its yoga and meditation classes.

People arrive from all over the world with serious health concerns to experience a structured support system of "pure living foods" that treats illnesses and diseases deemed to be "incurable" by Western allopathic medicine. "You've been robbed economically, you've been lied to, and you end up here," Hippocrates codirector Dr. Brian Clement tells new arrivals. "You either get here enlightened, or frightened."

During my three-week stay in the program I encountered people of all ages battling a range of deadly diseases—cancers, multiple sclerosis, Parkinson's, leukemia, diabetes. A Los Angeles real estate investor in his late fifties arrived with severe MS symptoms. I watched him the first week shuffle along slowly and stiffly on wobbly legs like someone trying to keep his balance on a storm-tossed ship. After two weeks on the diet he marched around with renewed vitality, showing no obvious symptoms of the disease. When his turn came to speak on Friday, the day each week that new graduates of the program can share their experiences with each other, he choked up with emotion and could only stammer "thank you" a few times before dissolving into tears.

Bonnie Lovett was a forty-nine-year-old periodic guest I interviewed who had been diagnosed with an aggressive form of brain tumors the previous year. She described for me how she drastically changed her eating habits until she only consumed wheatgreass juice, sprouts, and other raw living foods. She credits this Hippocrates regimen with saving her life. When she had another MRI scan of her brain in May 2005, it showed the tumors had vanished. She says physicians at the National Institutes of Health in Bethesda, Maryland, where she was tested, wrote the words "incredible" and "unbelievable" on her medical chart.

No one associated with Hippocrates made any public claims—at least that I heard—about being able to cure cancer or anything else. They only profess to provide an environment and a natural-foods strategy that empowers people to use their immune systems in their own wellness process. It just so happens that many of those coming here with serious illnesses are considered "throw-away" or "lost-cause" cases by practitioners of modern Western medicine, which makes their apparent recoveries at Hippocrates all the more impressive.

"Over the past decade we have been seeing younger and younger people here with brain cancers and leukemia. We are even seeing menopause symptoms in women who are in their twenties and thirties," explained Clement, who must be about sixty years of age but looks two decades younger. "There is no question that exposure to synthetic chemicals is the core reason for this increase in catastrophic illnesses."

The idea of pure food as medicine is taken quite literally here, and fresh wheatgrass juice is the food drink of choice. Less than two ounces of wheatgrass juice is said to be nutritionally equivalent to consuming nearly three pounds of fresh vegetables and 103 vitamins and minerals. Wheatgrass contains nature's richest source of chlorophyll and acts as a potent immune system booster, body-organ cleanser, and toxins neutralizer. The

Hippocrates program utilizes a mix of components that act synergistically with the wheatgrass. These include sprouted seeds and grains, raw uncooked vegetables, daily exercise, periodic fasting, colon cleansings to remove toxic-waste accumulations, taking supplements derived only from naturally occurring whole foods, and the cultivation of positive attitudes.

The secret of perfect health, says toxin specialist Dr. Sherry Rogers, "is in getting your body so chemically unloaded and nutrient primed, that it heals itself." That sums up what I observed and experienced in the Hippocrates program. To detox the chemicals out of my system, each day I drank four ounces of wheatgrass juice, took several dozen chlorella tablets (a green algae supplement), exercised for forty-five minutes on a stairclimber, then sat in an infrared sauna for as long as I could stand it. I also fasted for twenty-four hours every week and had several colon-cleansing sessions and three massages.

There's a compelling logic behind using a mix of saunas, fasting, and colon cleansing. Infrared saunas use less temperature than conventional saunas and produce twice the sweat volume. Their heat energy draws chemicals out of fat and excretes them as sweat. Mayo Clinic studies have demonstrated the value of using these saunas on congestive heart failure patients to improve heart function, doing so without the side effects of drug therapies. A toxicologist pointed out to me that it was Scientology founder L. Ron Hubbard who first wrote about using saunas to detox synthetic chemicals from body fat in the late 1970s, linking it to the benefits of bringing the body's biochemistry back into natural balance.

Periodic fasts help to stress cells in the body to secrete chemicals. An additional health benefit was documented at the National Institute on Aging, whose chief of neurosciences, Mark Mattson, has shown how intermittent fasts—either eating only every other day, or not eating for twenty-one hours straight each day—increases the production of proteins in the brain that foster the growth of new nerve cells. This apparently enables the brain to repair damage caused by synthetic chemicals and may prevent Alzheimer's, Parkinson's, and related disorders.

Colon cleansings are designed to rid our septic system of accumulated waste toxins. Whatever food waste that isn't digested or eliminated ends up being baked into the cells of our intestines at 100.2 degrees Fahren-

heit, the human intestinal temperature. Unless removed, this matter becomes a toxins magnet and increases the length of time these toxins remain in our bodies.

Medical science researchers are generating a wealth of data supporting
the Hippocrates philosophy of applying pure foods to health and healing.
At Britain's Institute of Food Research, a review of international nutritional research up to 2002 produced a study that concluded: "Evidence
that diet is a key environmental factor affecting the incidence of many
chronic diseases is overwhelming. The food we eat contains thousands of
biologically active substances, many of which have the potential to provide substantial health benefits."

This news summary of research exploring the impact of food on curing disease appeared on the *New Scientist* magazine Web site (November
27, 2005): "Eating a specific food supplement could permanently change
your behavior for the better, or reverse [disorders and] diseases such as
schizophrenia, Huntington's or cancer." While this claim "may sound like
science fiction," continued the article, "such treatments are looking increasingly plausible" based on recent medical studies showing how diet
can alter human DNA.

During my three-week stay in detox-land, this story appeared in
Britain's BBC News headlined, "High-veg Diet Wards Off Cancer." It
summarized a report from the medical journal *Cancer, Epidemiology, Biomarkers and Prevention* that revealed how "raw vegetables are more protective than cooked ones" in cutting the risk of pancreatic cancer by more
than half. The most highly protective raw veggies were identified as
onions, garlic, carrots, and dark leafy plants such as spinach and broccoli,
all staples of the Hippocrates program diet. "We found strong confirma-
tion that simple life choices can provide significant protection from cancer," wrote the study's authors.

The Detox Strategy Works

On my last day at Hippocrates, a nurse drew eight vials of blood and sent
them off with a urine sample to the Accu-Chem Laboratory in Dallas for
my second round of body burden testing. A week later the results were

mailed to me and I scheduled a phone consultation with Accu-Chem's CEO, Dr. John Laseter, so he could analyze my scores.

"Your detox had an impact," Laseter announced. "Your total chemical load dropped out of the picture."

Pesticides that had been detected at higher-than-average levels the first time were now negligible in my blood. But several compounds such as arsenic had almost doubled in concentration. Counterintuitively, it turns out this was good news because it meant the chemicals stored in body fat were being secreted into my bloodstream for an eventual cleansing by my liver.

By far, the greater concentrations of chemicals are stored in our body fat. Laseter explained to me that the ratio of chemical molecules of blood to fat is about 1 to 200 or more, depending on the type of chemical and the area of fat in the body. That means having four parts per billion of DDE pesticide in my blood reflected eight hundred or more parts per billion in my body fat. My detox had leached the pesticides from fat and blood faster than the heavy metals, so the higher levels of arsenic showing up in the second blood test indicated an ongoing detox of fat cells.

This revelation about body-fat contaminations contrasted with blood indicators made me realize how the widespread chemical blood testing conducted by the U.S. Centers for Disease Control and Prevention give us just a narrow picture of how truly polluted we have become. As our society has gotten more obese, we have been absorbing ever-greater concentrations of synthetic chemicals. The fatter we become the more we are transformed into chemical time bombs.

As if that wasn't disturbing enough Laseter added another insight that further complicates our dilemma. "The human body is like a sponge for chemicals. We bioaccumulate them in our fat. But once the chemicals enter the body they metabolize. You may ingest one or two compounds and you may end up with five or six more because your body metabolizes and creates new compounds."

As one of the world's leading experts in the field of biochemistry, with more than one hundred peer-reviewed scientific papers to his credit, Laseter is a cautious scientist whose words are carefully chosen. He was the first U.S. scientist to lecture before the entire European Union Parliament on the perils we face from our chemical body burdens, and for ten years he served on the Science Advisory Board of the United States Environmental Protection Agency. So when he uses the word "scary," as he did in conversation with me, to describe the challenges we confront from synthetic chemicals, it's time to shake off complacency and take urgent notice.

"Life has been here evolving on this planet in a mix of chemicals for four-and-a-half billion years," Laseter observed. "It's only in the last three or so generations of our species that we've introduced tens of thousands of new synthetic chemical compounds for us to absorb. In time maybe we can adapt to what we've created. But the more mixes we introduce and the more synergies we create, the more we will stress our physiology. There is a big risk involved. If you think about it, this starts to get really scary."

Where do we even begin to start in trying to protect ourselves? To that question Laseter had a ready answer. We can't blame authorities or institutions within the economy or government, or engage in finger-pointing of any sort, except perhaps while standing in front of a mirror. "It comes down to personal accountability," he told me. "We are responsible for ourselves."

A Commitment to Health

Human nature seems to dictate that we cherish our myths and protect them with ingeniously constructed self-deceptions. When those myths eventually shatter, we express anger and indignation, often followed by a renewed commitment to denial. An illustration of this cycle surfaced in a small Pennsylvania town during Christmas 2005, when a teacher casually mentioned to a class of six- and seven-year-olds that Santa Claus was a myth. Her timing and discretion in making this statement might be faulted, but what enraged parents even more than the myth being exposed was exposure of their complicity in perpetuating it.

Parents began phoning the school superintendent demanding the teacher's dismissal. News stories quoted the parents describing how distressed they felt when their children came home in tears and accused them of being liars. Every one of these adults vowed to re-indoctrinate their child with the falsehood that Santa Claus is a real person with magical powers, even devising elaborate deceptions such as leaving footprints of

Santa in the fireplace on Christmas morning. This relatively innocuous case of mythmaking provides a glimpse at the depth of emotion that can surface around the much more insidious myth at the center of the Hundred-Year Lie.

To what extent will we continue lying to ourselves and each other to evade the truth about our addiction to the synthetics mythology? Psychologists call denial a "natural" first reaction to any revelation that forces us to think about making drastic changes in our lives. As the old saying goes, we don't fix leaks in a roof when it isn't raining, especially if we've never experienced a rainstorm.

A chemical storm is upon us. The necessity to change our habits can no longer be covered up or denied. The challenge for those of us who recognize this threat is to exercise self-discipline.

"You're going to keep being seduced by what will kill you," Dr. Brian Clement warns graduates of the Hippocrates program as they are preparing to head home. He knows how difficult it is for most of us to remain self-disciplined about what we put in our bodies and on our bodies in the face of so many cultural temptations to remain lazy or gluttonous.

Our internal saboteur often triumphs because most of us are slaves to our food habits and our cravings for the conveniences of modern life. Habits of mind quickly develop into addictions of the body. The more intense our cravings for harmful foods the greater the likelihood we also possess—or will develop—biochemical deficiencies and imbalances. To break that vicious cycle requires a dramatic commitment to an entirely new way of being.

The lesson to be drawn from what I saw and experienced at Hippocrates is startling in its simplicity. Merely by choosing a diet of pure foods and a lifestyle free of synthetics, we can detoxify ourselves and initiate the healing of many degenerative illnesses and diseases.

Whether you put this lesson into practice is entirely dependent on your conscience and your willpower. We have all been complicit in perpetuating the Hundred-Year Lie, and some of us have personally profited from it. But given the trends detailed in this book, if the current system remains intact, we must ask what form of human being will be left to reflect on the fruits of this belief system?

We can either free ourselves of the Hundred-Year Lie, or we can choose by our inaction to continue buying into the myth. The decision is upon us. We no longer have the luxury of postponing it. If hundreds of millions of us make the choice to stop supporting the lie with our money and our lives, that unity can set in motion changes with the potential to make life and health on this planet once again sustainable.

9 PRACTICAL STEPS YOU CAN TAKE

1. Study the Labels—On every product with an ingredient label, whether it be food, medicine, or household items, familiarize yourself with the chemical names by comparing them to a list of toxins you have compiled based on information in this book and at www.hundredyearlie.com. The more toxins you identify in a product the more determined you should be to reject buying it.

2. Replace Home Pesticides—A wide range of natural, non-toxic remedies exists for common household pests. The neem tree from India provides a natural insecticide for plants and gardens, while oil of peppermint spray works for ants, and baking soda mixed with powdered sugar helps to repel cockroaches.

3. Drink Wheatgrass Juice—To help strengthen your immune system and cleanse your body of chemical toxins, drink wheatgrass juice every day, or at least whenever you can. Inquire at health food stores or do an online search for the most convenient places in your area to purchase fresh wheatgrass, or to learn how to grow and juice your own.

4. Do Intermittent Fasting—By eating only every other day, or, at the very least, doing a juice fast one day a week, you stress the cells of your body in a manner that aids its secretion of chemical toxins from body tissues and organs. Periodic fasting will also help you recognize the range and severity of your food dependencies.

5. Detox with Saunas—When combined with vigorous exercise, saunas can aid your body in squeezing out in sweat the more deeply embedded chemical toxins. Ideally, find a "far infrared sauna" to use, which creates less heat than

conventional saunas but produces twice the sweat volume. Natural, not synthetic, mineral supplements, such as niacin, calcium, zinc, and magnesium, should be considered after each sauna use if you aren't consuming wheatgrass regularly.

6. Eat Organic Foods—Whenever and wherever you can, purchase organic foods and eat at organic food restaurants. The pesticide residues on these foods will be much lower than nonorganics, and you should find many fewer synthetic chemicals of all kinds contaminating organic brands. You will also be supporting the organic foods industry and making a statement with every purchase.

7. Choose Nutritious Organics—Consuming these raw foods three or more times a week will support your liver's detox functions and produce immune agents in your body to fight infection: broccoli, garlic, spinach, cabbage, sprouts, blueberries, ginger, and curcumin.

8. Compile a Personal Toxins List—Write out a list of synthetic chemicals you consume each day from your foods, medications, and personal-care products. Post the list somewhere prominently in your home. Make a conscious effort to limit your intake of these chemicals. Make a choice to live a toxin-free life and monitor your progress by recruiting like-minded people into support groups.

9. Read and Sign the Declaration—At the Web site for this book, www.hundredyearlie.com, you will find the Declaration of Interdependence. This statement of principle will be presented to the United Nations secretary general on behalf of the citizens of the world to show a unified determination to reverse our dependence on synthetic chemicals. Please sign the Declaration posted on the Web site and encourage your friends and family to do the same.

HOW TO DETOXIFY YOURSELF

If you want to discover the extent of your own chemical body burden, or that carried by your child, testing is available from reputable labs. You can also undergo a detox program at a specialty health center to rid yourself of the body burden or to treat a serious health condition. The following sources are a good place to start.

Detoxification Books and Self-Help Resources

Toxic Overload, by Paula Baillie-Hamilton

Paula Baillie-Hamilton is a British M.D. who also has a doctorate in human metabolism from the University of Oxford. In this book Baillie-Hamilton explains how chemicals in pesticides, plastics, cosmetics, cleaning solvents, and many other products commonly used in our daily lives accumulate to toxic levels in our bodies and break down our natural defenses against disease. Of particular interest is her three-step program to a chemical-free life. She proposes specific forms of supplementation, as well as the "7-day De-Sludge Diet," and dispenses practical advice on everything from how to achieve a chemical-free home to chemical-free beauty products.

The Body Restoration Plan, by Paula Baillie-Hamilton

Considering the magnitude of the fat epidemic that is sweeping industrialized nations, the relationship between synthetic chemicals and weight management is an obvious topic of interest. Applying her research in chemical toxicity to the very practical and results-driven field of weight loss, Baillie-Hamilton argues that the human body will benefit from a powerful, naturally occurring weight-regulation system, if only we stop damaging it with toxic hormone-altering chemicals found in our everyday lives.

The Detox Solution, by Patricia Fitzgerald

Patricia Fitzgerald's credentials include a master's degree in Chinese medicine and a doctorate in homeopathic medicine. Fitzgerald fully explains detoxification in this practical guide. She divides her coverage into three sections. In part one, readers become aware of the range of toxins and then are given ideas on how to replace or avoid them. In part two, they learn how the body naturally detoxifies and the ways these processes are compromised by toxicity. Part three moves on to methods of supporting our detox processes and of building a high state of well-being.

Our Toxic World, by Doris J. Rapp

Doris Rapp is a pediatric allergist and environmental medical physician whose book *Our Toxic World* practically addresses the hazards of our modern world by teaching how to recognize health-related signs in your body associated with particular products and chemicals. Rapp draws from a wide range of meticulously detailed references and tells the story of how chemicals damage your body, brain, and behavior. She is eager for you to figure out where and when you were exposed, helping you document your suspicions about harmful exposures, and enabling you to consider what you and your doctor can do about them together.

Detoxify or Die, by Sherry A. Rogers

Sherry A. Rogers is a leading environmental medicine authority who covers just about everything you would ever want to know about exposure to chemical toxins and strategies for detoxifying your body. In clear, nontechnical language she explains various laboratory and home-testing approaches to determining your body burden of chemicals, and provides information on saunas and other programs for lightening the load. The resource guide at the end of this book provides a wealth of guidance.

Physician Resources

If your research has led you to the conclusion that you want to get tested for your chemical body burden or find out if your suspicions are accurate about links between your symptoms and products you use, you'll first want to find a physician who can help you.

Environmental Medicine:
American Academy of Environmental Medicine, http://www.aaem.com
Environmental medicine physician locator,
http://www.aaem.com/referable_physicians.htm

Functional Medicine:
The Institute for Functional Medicine,
http://www.functionalmedicine.org
Functional medicine physician locator,
http://www.functionalmedicine.org/findfmphysician/form.asp

Toxicity-Testing Laboratories

Diagnostic laboratories are typically accessed with a physician's referral, and they specify which of the sometimes hundreds of tests to complete. Typically, a kit is mailed to you, which your physician can then use to fulfill the sampling requirements (often in the form of saliva, blood, or urine). The sample is then sealed and certified by the physician, and then mailed back to the lab for analysis and results. Costs are significant, so testing is a serious proposition designed to assist you in evaluating a health practice that could radically change the quality of your life. Reporting is confidential.

Great Smokies Diagnostics Laboratory, http://www.gsdl.com
Great Smokies Diagnostic Laboratory has helped pioneer the field of laboratory functional testing. Functional testing assesses the dynamic inter-

relationship of physiological systems, thereby creating a more complete picture of one's health, unlike traditional allopathic testing, which is more concerned about the pathology of disease.

Immunosciences Lab, http://www.immuno-sci-lab.com
As one of the pioneering laboratories in the field of molecular medicine, Immunosciences Lab analyzes complex diseases that directly or indirectly involve the human immune system. Through its unique diagnostic testing, the lab provides physicians with tools to inhibit disease progression and perhaps ultimately prevent certain occurrences. ISL offers more than four hundred tests.

Accu-Chem Laboratories, http://www.accuchem.com
Accu-Chem Laboratories is a clinical and forensic toxicology laboratory that provides diagnostic testing for a wide array of environmental and occupational toxins. The test panels that Accu-Chem offers include some of the most common and persistent chemical compounds the average person may encounter: chlorinated pesticides, chlordane, organophosphorous pesticide metabolites, aromatic volatile solvents, brominated volatile solvents, heavy metal analysis, pyrethroids, pthalate metabolites, permethrins, formaldehyde/formic acid panel, and more.

Detoxification Programs and Centers

Hippocrates Health Institute, http://www.hippocratesinst.com
The Hippocrates Health Institute has been a leader in the field of natural and alternative health care and education since 1956. The Hippocrates philosophy is dedicated to the belief that a pure, enzyme-rich diet, complemented by positive thinking and noninvasive therapies, is an essential element on the path to optimum health.

Environmental Health Center–Dallas, http://www.ehcd.com
The Environmental Health Center–Dallas addresses health and disease as they relate to the environment. With a staff of more than seventy, including physicians, surgeons, scientists, nutritionists, and physical therapists,

the center provides full-service medical care with a special emphasis on the impact of environmental factors. According to William J. Rea, who founded the clinic in 1974, various exposures may cause sleep disturbance; learning disorders; blood vessel, colon, and bladder inflammations; as well as a host of other inflammatory problems. The "environment" involves all of our surroundings, including everything we breathe, eat, or touch. The center offers a six-day-per-week, physician-supervised program.

Tree of Life Rejuvenation Center, www.treeoflife.nu, 866-394-2520
Utilizing ideas developed in the book *Spiritual Nutrition* by Gabriel Cousens, M.D., this retreat facility in southern Arizona, near the border of Mexico, offers ten-day detox packages along with fasting retreats and workshops on organic vegan food as medicine.

OTHER USEFUL RESOURCES

Organic Consumers Association, www.organicconsumers.org
This nationwide organization of nearly one million members is dedicated to preserving pure organic standards for food and other products.

Naturally Occurring Standards Group, www.nosg.org
A non-profit group campaigning to create a naturally occurring standard (NOS), as advocated in this book, to clearly separate on labels the synthetic vitamins and minerals from products derived exclusively from plant-based sources.

MODERN SCIENCE AFFIRMS ANCIENT CURES

Our rediscovery of ancient healing wisdom, typically called folk remedies, and using the laboratory tools of modern science are revolutionizing our understanding of the naturally occurring food, herbal, and plant treatments. What Western medicine really seems to be rediscovering is its own traditional wisdom roots. The founding father of modern medicine, Hippocrates, the ancient Greek in whose name all new physicians in the United States swear an oath, was himself a practitioner and teacher of Unani Tibb, the traditional medicine of the Middle East in the ancient world.

Every civilization and tribal culture that perpetuated itself in any form up to the present day maintained some structure of traditional medicine based on the healing properties of plants, shrubs, and trees native to its land. Through trial and error and intuition each society over the generations isolated and codified lists of botanicals that either worked individually or in synergistic combinations with proven healing powers for a wide range of illnesses and diseases. That entire collective body of accumulated knowledge was mostly discarded as irrelevent by Western countries during the twentieth century in their mad rush of enthusiasm to embrace the "scientific method" and the synthetics paradigm.

Traditional medicines and the ancient wisdom traditions that utilized them have always been based upon observations about the laws of nature. For a list of illnesses and diseases for which medical science has affirmed ancient cures, go to www.hundredyearlie.com.

MORE EVIDENCE TO PENETRATE OUR DENIAL

Since publication of the hardcover edition of *The Hundred-Year Lie* only one year ago, a wealth of science studies and medical research has emerged showing even more clearly how truly vulnerable we all are to the on-slaught of synthetic chemical toxins, and providing support for many of the key contentions and findings presented in this book.

The Hundred-Year Lie received widespread media attention when it ap-peared. *The New York Post* devoted an entire newspaper page to some of the book's findings, while I made appearances on the ABC morning show *The View*, on the Fox network's *Fox & Friends* morning show, and on fifty-five radio interview programs. Because of the book's message about the impact of chemicals on longevity, I was invited to speak before the 14th Annual International Congress on Anti-Aging Medicine in Las Ve-gas, attended by several thousand physicians and medical researchers. For-eign publication rights to the book were sold in China, South Korea, Taiwan, and Holland.

Despite this attention the book seemed to have a negligible impact on public awareness. Understandably, both global warming and the war in Iraq had taken center stage. But there were other deeper reasons, in my opinion. The book became an object lesson exposing the layers of denial that we are capable of exhibiting when confronted with inconvenient truths about the repercussions of our lifestyle choices. It is far easier and re-assuring to reflexively dismiss a message as simple scare-mongering than to examine its authenticity through the lens of our own naked vulnerability.

The litany of revelatory headlines, however, will not go away and over the past year provided a grim reminder of the accumulating perils we face in the long-term:

"Toxins Create Hermaphrodite Polar Bears" (*The Independent*, UK, 1/10/06)

"Report Raises Flag on Fluoride" (*USA Today*, 3/22/06)

"Drug Firms Inventing Diseases" (BBC News, 4/11/06)

"U.S. Has Second Worst Newborn Death Rate in Modern World" (CNN, 5/9/06)

"Plastics Link to 'Macho' Female Mice" (*New Scientist*, 5/14/06)

"Common Plastic Linked to Prostate Cancer" (*Los Angeles Times*, 6/1/06)

"Use of Antipsychotics by the Young Rose Fivefold" (*The New York Times*, 6/6/06)

"Study Links Autism, Pollution" (*Los Angeles Times*, 6/23/06)

"China's Growing Pollution Reaches U.S." (AP, 7/28/06)

"Food Chemicals May Harm Humans" (BBC News, 9/21/06)

"Mercury Contamination Moves Beyond Fish" (ABC News, 10/18/06)

"UN: Number of Ocean 'Dead Zones' Rise" (AP, 10/19/06)

"Chemical Pollution Harms Children's Brains" (*The Independent*, UK, 11/8/06)

"Plastics Poisoning World's Seas" (BBC News, 12/7/06)

Mainstream magazines also weighed in with in-depth articles on the threat to health posed by the body burdens of synthetic chemicals that we all carry. In the October 2006 issue of *National Geographic,* twenty-eight pages were devoted to "The Pollution Within," with the author of the article, science writer David Ewing Duncan, revealing how his blood test looking for 320 chemicals had detected 165, some at alarmingly high levels. Flame retardant chemicals in him, for instance, were measured in the toxic range and a toxicologist speculated that Duncan had been contaminated from contact with flame retardants that coat airplane passenger seats.

Duncan quoted toxicologists as saying that "dose is everything" and that "minuscule smidgens of chemicals inside us are mostly nothing to

worry about." Then he proceeded to challenge those arguments by pointing out how certain illnesses over the past few decades have been "rising
mysteriously." Autism has increased tenfold, leukemia is up 62 percent, a
doubling of male birth defects, childhood brain cancer is up 40 percent,
etc. Again and again, Duncan quoted experts as admitting "we don't have
the data in humans to know if the current levels [of chemicals in the
body] are safe." He also cited the potential dangers of "chemical cocktails," mixtures of chemicals that may do "little harm on their own but act
together to damage human cells."

To illustrate the range of science developments in the year since this
book's initial publication, here are some examples of where the new findings are in alignment with this book:

**Book contention: Wastewater treatment and water purification
plants cannot remove many common synthetic chemicals and as a result, both humans and wildlife are experiencing health consequences
that may include genetic and reproductive abnormalities.**

A significant and unprecedented collection of forty science studies appeared in the American Chemical Society journal, *Environmental Science &
Technology*, which devoted its entire December 2006 issue to the "effects
of emerging contaminants on people and planet." These studies col-
lectively reveal how wastewater treatment and water purification plants
throughout the industrialized world are recycling huge quantities and varieties of synthetic chemicals into the environment because the removal
technology is not sophisticated enough to eliminate designer toxins.

Below is a summary of just a few of those forty studies:

- A study of North American rainwater at four northeastern U.S.
  sites and two sites in southern Canada found significantly high
  concentrations of PFOAs, which are used as stain-resistant coatings on paper, particularly fast food packaging. The main source
  of this contamination seemed to be the urban corridor between
  New York and Washington, D.C.
- Carbon filters on water treatment plants often fail to remove
  PFOAs and PFOSs, both types of perfluorinated surfactants
  found in consumer products. Both the Moehre and Ruhr rivers

in Germany were found to be contaminated, apparently because food industry sewage sludge had been spread on farm fields near the rivers. Drinking water taken from these rivers had alarmingly high levels of these chemicals.

- Flame retardants (PBDEs) in the bodies of North Americans are ten times higher than anywhere else in the world. These retardants are absorbed by fish and bioaccumulate up the food chain into humans.

- Dozens of types of disinfectant chemical by-products were detected at twelve drinking water treatment plants, including twenty-eight "new previously unidentified disinfection by-products."

- Two common "complexing agents" called BT and TT, used in dishwasher detergents and as anti-corrosives, escape removal in wastewater treatment plants and bioaccumulate in the environment. A study of seven rivers in Switzerland found concentrations of both contaminants.

- A study of surface waters in Germany and Switzerland found that certain types of barbiturates, whose production was halted decades ago, still pollute the environment and resist breakdown.

- Organic wastewater contaminants were identified and analyzed from solid waste produced by wastewater treatment plants in seven U.S. states. This waste was spread on farm fields. In any one sample taken, up to forty-five chemical contaminants were found out of eighty-seven that were being sought, which means the actual numbers of chemical contaminants surviving wastewater treatment will be in the hundreds if not thousands. Biosolids are "highly enriched" with these contaminants, said the study authors, and the results "demonstrate the need" to better determine the health risks, since 50 percent of biosolids produced in the United States are spread on lands, many of which support crops.

- Two chemical compounds used in cancer chemotherapy and the treatment of autoimmune diseases were found to survive treated wastewater processes and to persist in groundwater with unknown toxic effects on aquatic life.

- Wastewater from thirty on-site treatment systems in two Colorado counties—Summit and Jefferson—was analyzed for organic wastewater contaminants. Of the twenty-four target chemical compounds, 88 percent were detected in the samples. Some compounds, such as endocrine disrupting chemicals, disinfectants, antimicrobial agents, and pharmaceuticals, were found in every sample.
- Aircraft deicer and anti-icer fluid runoff creates endocrine disruption and toxicity in aquatic life, but scientists are having difficulty studying the effects because trade secrecy laws enable manufacturers to hide toxic chemical ingredients from public view and as a result, "much of the toxicity is due to unidentified additives," concluded the scientists involved in this study.

A missing piece of the puzzle about the health effects of these chemicals being released into the environment was provided by U.S. Geological Survey studies and revealed in *The Washington Post*, which published a front-page article on September 6, 2006, describing the test results from rivers in the Washington, D.C., area. These rivers provide the tap water for several million residents of D.C., northern Virginia, and suburban Maryland.

At least 80 percent of all bass caught in those rivers and river tributaries were found to have intersex reproductive organs, with the males growing eggs in their testes. Since 2003, when these abnormalities in fish were first discovered in the upper Potomac River and in West Virginia, the incidence of intersex births has spread rapidly and widely.

Hormone disrupting chemicals released by wastewater treatment plants into these rivers were identified as the probable culprits for these abnormalities. The problem may be "a result of several pollutants acting in combination," according to the study authors. In other words, chemical synergies or the additive effects of chemicals acting on each other may be producing these mutant strains of fish.

Even though the U.S. Congress directed the U.S. Environmental Protection Agency in 1996 to develop a screening program to identify which chemicals are causing abnormalities, a decade later *not a single chemical* has been tested by the EPA. Officials at that agency confessed that the technological challenge was simply too overwhelming.

Scientists interviewed by *The Washington Post* expressed shock and dismay at this spread of hormone disrupting chemicals and the complete inability of the EPA to even study the problem. As for the possible threat to human health that exposure to tap water may pose, a spokesman for the area's water utility confessed that they have no idea whether water purification plants can remove the mutation-causing chemicals before humans ingest the water. "We don't even know if we are analyzing the water to look for the right things," revealed Charles Murray, general manager of the Fairfax (Virginia) Water utility.

Four months after this article appeared, the U.S. Geological Survey reported finding still a third species of fish in the Potomac River basin that had developed intersex characteristics. A scientist with the agency, Vicki Blazer, also linked these reproductive abnormalities to large-scale fish kills that began occurring in the region in 2002, in which fish with suppressed immune systems developed lesions and died. Synthetic chemical contaminants in the water were cited as the probable cause for this destruction of immune cells and disease resistance.

Book contention: Synthetic chemical synergies and additive effects are emerging as a global threat to human and animal life.

Scientific American magazine published an article in May 2006 titled, "Mixing It Up: Harmless Levels of Chemicals Prove Toxic Together," and cited several new science studies that constitute "a growing body of work showing that chemicals in combination can produce a wide range of effects even at low concentrations." Pesticides and phthalates—chemical softners used to make plastics flexible—were two compounds noted as having some of the more powerful observed effects when mixed.

"These findings on mixtures pose an incredible challenge for regulators," continued the article. "With tens of thousands of chemicals in regular use worldwide, assessing which combination might prove harmful is a gargantuan task." Given today's limited budgetary resources and technology, the article could have added that the task is impossible and the potential threats to human health are beyond measure.

In an overview of recent science studies on cancer, Dr. Devra Davis, a professor of epidemiology at the University of Pittsburgh's Graduate School of Health, writing in a February 2007 issue of *Newsweek* magazine (and circulated again by MSNBC), made a case that the synergistic and additive effects of synthetic chemicals acting together should be a growing cause for alarm. Wrote Dr. Davis: "There's plenty of solid human evidence that combined pollutants can cause more harm together than they do alone." She lists numerous examples, such as childhood cancers occurring in children with no inherited risk of the disease, and rising rates of lung cancer in women with no exposure to smoking.

Professor Davis went on to warn that we all have become guinea pigs in a vast chemical experiment. "There's a problem with the way the United States and other countries look at toxicity in commercial agents. Regulators nowadays often won't take action until enough people have already complained of harm. This makes little sense . . . people have a right to know whether products they use on themselves and their children contain compounds that increase their risk of disease. They also have a right to expect that government will prevent companies from selling products that are harmful to children. To do otherwise is to treat our children like lab rats in a vast uncontrollable experiment."

Our body burdens of synthetic chemical exposures over a lifetime should be a cause for concern said Dr. Davis: "We're beginning to realize that the sum total of a person's exposure to all the little amounts of cancerous agents in the environment may be just as harmful as big doses of a few well-known carcinogens. Our chances of getting cancer reflect the full gamut of carcinogens we're exposed to each day—in air, water, and food pollution and in cancerous ingredients or contaminants in household cleaners, clothing, furniture, and the dozens of personal care products many of us use daily."

Book contention: Synthetic chemicals contribute to the incidence of violence, depression, and other behavioral disorders, especially in children.

A food additive found in most fast foods and junk foods may trigger violence and depression later in life if the fetus absorbs its mother's toxic habits. That conclusion came from research conducted at the National Institutes of Health outside Washington, D.C., which has turned up persuasive evidence that junk food diets can cause depression, violence, and other antisocial behaviors.

A group of eighty volunteers, many of them with criminal records of violence, went through a double-blind study in which half had their omega-6 fatty acids (found in fast foods and junk foods) drastically reduced and replaced with more healthy omega-3 fatty acids as found primarily in fish oil. The result was a startling drop in anger, aggression, and depression.

The clinician in charge of the study, Dr. Joseph Hibbein, said our modern diets are "changing the very architecture and functioning of the brain." The key finding of the NIH research is that omega-6 fatty acids, found in everything from margarine and ice cream to snack foods such as potato chips, have replaced the healthy omega-3s and produced severe disruptions of serotonin and dopamine in the brains of junk food addicts. Low serotonin is known to be linked to depression, the risk of suicide, and violent and impulsive behaviors. Dopamine is crucial to decision-making.

When these deficiencies occur as the human brain is in rapid development—as a fetus, in the first five years of life, and at puberty—the brain's architecture can be permanently altered. That means a mother's diet while pregnant can help predict whether her child will grow up to suffer depression or be prone to antisocial acts. Dr. Hibbein and other researchers have compared statistics of omega-6 consumption since the 1960s in thirty-eight industrialized countries to the increase in murder rates in those countries during the same period. They are a perfect match! These toxic changes in our diets, Dr. Hibbein told Britain's *Guardian* on October 17, 2006, "are a very large uncontrolled experiment that may have contributed to the societal burden of aggression, depression, and cardiovascular death."

"Chemical Impairment of Children's Brains Declared a 'Pandemic,' " read some newspaper headlines when *The Lancet,* one of the four leading medical journals in the world, published a study by a team of scientists from the Harvard School of Public Health in November 2006 that identified 201 chemicals found in everyday use as being responsible for impairing children's brain development, lowering their IQs, shortening their attention spans, and triggering behavioral problems. "The combined evidence suggests that neurodevelopmental disorders caused by industrial chemicals have created a silent pandemic in modern society," wrote the study authors, who estimated that one in six of all children now display developmental disabilities as a result of exposure to these chemicals that range from phthalates and Bisphenol A found in the lining of canned food, to methylmercury, PCBs, and in the ingredients in cleaning fluids, glues, cosmetics, and pesticides.

Some toxicologists publicly ridiculed *The Lancet* study and its authors as engaging in "scare-mongering" and being "overly alarmist" in describing the chemical exposure health effects as a pandemic. Other skeptics took the approach of describing our body burdens of these chemicals as being at such low doses that we can consider their presence inside of us as "normal."

Medicine and science are constantly trying to redefine what is normal in a way that warps our awareness of the dangers we face, says the cancer researcher, Dr. Devra Davis, who notes how in response to the growing numbers of young girls with breasts, the certifying board for pediatric endocrinology has changed its recommendation of what is natural and normal. "We believe this is a dangerous move," wrote Dr. Davis. "If we say that it's now normal for young girls to develop breasts at ages 6 and 7, we will fail to pick up serious diseases that could account for this. We will also lose the chance to learn whether widely used agents in the environment, like those found in personal care products today or others that may enter the food supply, lay behind some of these patterns."

Book contention: Animal studies have not proven reliable indicators of synthetic chemical impacts on human health and as a result, thousands of experiments showing chemicals to be "safe" for consumer products are in doubt.

What if everything that medical science thought it knew based on laboratory testing of animals turned out to be wrong? A third reason for holding this point of view has emerged to be added to my original two reasons—that lab animals metabolize chemicals differently than humans, and lab tests using one chemical at a time cannot duplicate a real world environment in which humans are subjected to hundreds of chemicals simultaneously every day.

In 2006 it was discovered that a hidden variable affecting the outcomes of millions of experiments has been the standard diet given laboratory rodents, food that contained high levels of hormones. Mice and rats used in lab experiments have traditionally been fed soy as a key source of protein. Since at least 1931 it has been known that soy contains estrogen-like chemicals called phytoestrogens, but only now have scientists considered the extent to which these estrogens can skew test results. The chemicals disrupt natural hormone levels in animals much as they do in humans, disrupting normal growth and metabolism development, all of which can render invalid any studies that investigate the effects of synthetic chemicals on hormones, or differences between males and females in contracting diseases.

Dr. Julius Thigpen, a microbiologist at the National Institute of Environmental Health Sciences, was one of the first to sound the alarm after fellow scientists were unable to repeat some experiments and produce the same results. He investigated and found the lab animal diet was causing the variations. He reported his findings to a scientific journal, but his paper was rejected "because they didn't think it was important."

Other scientists tested the rodent food and came up with similar aberrant results and soon a revolution in thinking was underway. "This is a major problem," a biologist at Vanderbilt University Medical Center confessed to *The Dallas Morning News*. At the University of Colorado, Leslie Leinwand, a molecular biologist, publicly bemoaned how "we can't go back and do 20 years of experiments all over again."

Have We Become Like Ancient Romans?

What we may be witnessing is the repeat of a historical pattern of chemical contamination that generates its own peculiar state of public denial. One explanation given by historians for the decline of the Roman Empire involves the ruling class having slowly poisoned itself by absorbing lead, which was a metal widely used in cooking pots, utensils, wine urns, water pipes, and cosmetics.

Rulers such as Caligula and Nero, so this theory goes, went insane from absorbing lead. Infertility and lowered intelligence were among the many symptoms of lead toxicity. Lead use continued among the ruling classes despite their knowledge that it was toxic to the slaves who were forced to mine it.

Today the toxins we are exposed to may be much more varied and their effects much more complex—and thus subject to debate—but our state of denial about the health threat still resembles the Roman experience. We absorb thousands of synthetic chemicals during a lifetime and yet we look around us puzzled that so many illnesses and diseases have become epidemics.

We see firsthand or we read about the increased incidence of behavioral and mood disorders among our children, yet we want to deny that fast food and junk food chemicals can cause mental instability and violence. We hear about the genetic and reproductive mutations in wildlife caused by exposure to synthetic chemical combinations, particularly in water, yet we deny that anything similar can occur, or is occurring, within our own species.

We deny because we have become addicted to the conveniences of modern life, just as the ancient Romans became complacent about their lifestyle addictions that proved toxic to their health.

We deny because our arrogance blinds us to the lessons of history.

We deny because we choose to believe that we are too wise to be so foolish.

—Randall Fitzgerald
March 23, 2007

BIBLIOGRAPHY

Introduction: What Are We Doing to Ourselves?

Associated Press, "Colo. Scientists Find Chemicals in Waters," http://www.start.earth link.net, January 19, 2005

Baillie-Hamilton, Paula. *Toxic Overload.* Penguin, 2005.

Borenstein, Seth. "Traces of Toxic Chemicals Found in Supermarket Food." Knight-Ridder Newspapers, September 2, 2004.

Colborn, Theo; Dumanoski, Dianne; and Myers, John. *Our Stolen Future.* Plume, 1997.

Corning, Peter. *Nature's Magic.* Cambridge University Press, 2003.

Geitner, Paul. "Europeans Found to Eat Less Bad Fats Than Americans." *San Francisco Chronicle,* September 2, 2004.

Heilprin, John. "Flame Retardant Found in Lake Michigan." *Associated Press,* November 24, 2004.

Jowit, Juliette. "Pollutants Cause Huge Rise in Brain Diseases," *Observer,* August 15, 2004.

National Academies. "Major Advances in Biology Should Be Used to Assess Birth Defects From Toxic Chemicals." www4.nationalacademies.org, June 1, 2000.

Nestle, Marion. *Food Politics.* University of California Press, 2002.

Schlosser, Eric. *Fast Food Nation.* HarperCollins, 2002.

Skenazy, Lenore. "Fed up with the food industry," *The Press Democrat,* August 28, 2004.

Williams, Sally and Brindley, Madeleine. "The toxins that should alarm us all," *Western Mail,* UK, October 8, 2004.

Chapter One: Reading the Signs

American Chemistry Council: News & Media. "Biomonitoring," http://www.accnews media.com

Associated Press. "Experts Refute Anti-Bacterial Soap Claims," October 20, 2005.

Baillie-Hamilton, Paula. *Toxic Overload.* Penguin, 2005.

BiomonitoringInfo.org

Bridges, Betty. "Fragrance: Emerging Health and Environmental Concerns." *Flavour and Fragrance Journal,* 2002.

Carson, Rachel. *Silent Spring.* Mariner Books, 1962.

Coming Clean. "What is Body Burden?" http://chemicalbodyburden.org

Cone, Marla. "Federal Study Finds Human Bodies Loaded With Toxic Compounds." *Los Angeles Times,* July 22, 2005.

_____ "Report: EPA Failing to Study Chemicals' Health Risks." *Los Angeles Times,* July 13, 2005.

_____ *Silent Snow.* Grove Press, 2005.

Connor, Steve. "Geneticists Protest at DNA of Rice Becoming a Trade Secret," *Independent,* March 18, 2002.

CorpWatch.org Environmental Media Services. "Scientists Challenge New Study on Low Dose Effects of Toxic Chemicals," http://www.ems.org, February 13, 2003.

Environmental Working Group. "BodyBurden Fact Sheets." http://www.ewg.org/reports/bodyburdenchemicalindustryarchives.org

_____ "Anniston, Alabama."

_____ "Fact and Fiction."

_____ "FDA Warns Industry to Follow Law on Untested Ingredients," http://www.ewg.org/issues/cosmetics, March 7, 2005.

_____ "Killing the Right-to-Know."

_____ "PR (Public Relations)."

_____ "Responsible Care."

_____ "3M and Scotchgard."

_____ "Trade Secrets: The Inside Story," *Earth Island Journal* (http://earthisland.org), vol. 16, no. 4, Winter 2001–2002.

Epstein, Samuel. "PBS: Trade Secrets You Were Never Supposed to See," Cancer Prevention Coalition, March 23, 2001.

Fairechild, Diana. "Skypoxia," *The Jet Smart Newsletter,* March 27, 2004.

Fischer, Douglas. "The Body Burden," ANG Newspapers, March 16, 2005.

Great Smokies Diagnostic Lab. "Toxic Element Exposure Profile," http://www.gsdl.com

"How Toxic Is Your Bathroom?" http://www.independent.co.uk, October 24, 2005.

Kamrin, Michael. "Biomonitoring Basics." Environmental Health Research Foundation, June 2004.

_____ "Traces of Environmental Chemicals in the Human Body: Are They a Risk to Health?" American Council on Science and Health (http://www.acsh.org), May 1, 2003.

Krimsky, Sheldon. *Hormonal Chaos*. Johns Hopkins University Press, 2000.

Mayeda, Julie. "Contaminated Arctic Only Looks Pristine." *San Francisco Chronicle*, May 22, 2005.

National Environmental Trust. "Toxic Chemicals Widespread in Consumer Products," http://net.org, July 14, 2004.

National Institute of Environmental Health Sciences (http://www.niehs.nih.gov).

_____ "Epidemiology: Studying Disease Rates."

_____ "Our Chemical World, and Our Dilemma."

_____ "Susceptibility: The 'Why Me' Question."

National Pesticide Telecommunications Network. "Inert or Other Ingredients," http://nptn.orst.edu and http://www.ourstolenfuture.org

PBS: Trade Secrets (http://pbs.org/tradesecrets)

_____ "Audit Privilege Secrets."

_____ "Children at Risk."

_____ "Fighting Right-to-Know."

_____ "Hairspray."

_____ "Individuals."

_____ "Money and Politics."

_____ "Non-Disclosure."

_____ "PR Strategies."

_____ "Regulatory War."

_____ "Responses to Industry Comments."

_____ "Secrecy."

_____ "Voluntary Testing."

"The Poison Paradox," *National Geographic*, May 2005.

Price, Rabbi Gavriel. "Food Ingredients Labels: A Primer on Regulations," Daf Haskashrus, June & July 2003.

Public Employees for Environmental Responsibility. " 'Scotchgard' Whistleblower Files Federal Free Speech Lawsuit," http://www.ems.org, August 18, 2005.

Rapp, Doris J. *Our Toxic World*. Environmental Medical Research Foundation, 2004.

Sankey, John. "Why Science Can't Prove a Pesticide Is Safe," Pesticide Education Network.

Schafer, Kristin S.; Reeves, Margaret; Spitzer, Skip; and Kegley, Susan E. "Chemical Trespass," Pesticide Action Network, May 2004.

Simmons, Ralph A.; Grau, Karen A.C.; and Soffa, JoAnna R. "Keeping Secrets: Laws Protecting Confidential Business Information Are Open to Interpretation." http://packaginglaw.com, February 2003.

"Tests Reveal Chemical Cocktail in EU Minister's Blood: WWF." *Agence France Presse*, October 19, 2004.

Trautmann, Nancy. "The Dose Makes the Poison—Or Does It?" http://www.actionbio science.org

Walter, Martha L.; Kamrin, Michael A.; and Katz, Delores J. "Reporting on Risk, A Journalist's Handbook on Environmental Risk Assessment" (http:www.facsnet.org), February 14, 2000.

Williams, Rose Marie. "More on 'inerts,'" *Townsend Letter for Doctors and Patients,* July 2004.

Chapter Two: From the Womb to the Grave

Alexander, Richard. "Chemically Induced Diseases: Synergistic Effects and Cumulative Injuries caused by Toxic Chemicals—Understanding the Gulf War Syndrome and Multiple Chemical Sensitivity," http://www.consumerlawpage.com

Baillie-Hamilton, Paula. *Toxic Overload.* Penguin, 2005.

Bischoff, Erik. "Chemical Sensitivity in Symptomatic Cambodia Veterans." *Archives of Environmental Health,* December 2003.

Colborn, Theo; Dumanoski, Dianne; and Myers, John. *Our Stolen Future.* Plume, 1997.

Cone, Marla. "Hot on Parkinson's Trail," *Los Angeles Times,* November 27, 2005.

"Household Chemicals in Direct Link to Asthma Rise," *Times of London,* December 23, 2004.

Kolata, Gina. "Environment and Cancer: The Links Are Elusive," *The New York Times,* December 13, 2005.

Krimsky, Sheldon. *Hormonal Chaos.* Johns Hopkins University Press, 2000.

Lawrence, Felicity. "Combining food additives may be harmful," *The Guardian* (UK), December 21, 2005.

"Many Dangerous Chemicals in European Blood." *Reuters,* October 6, 2005.

Monosson, Emily. "Chemical Mixtures: Considering the Evolution of Toxicology and Chemical Assessment," *Environmental Health Perspectives,* vol. 113, no. 4, April 2005.

Moore, Kirk. "Brick Families Still Seek Answers on Autism," *Asbury Park Press,* February 1, 2005.

"Multiple chemical sensitivity," http://en.wikipedia.org

"New Car Smell Could Be Dangerous," ABC Good Morning America, September 27, 2005.

Our Stolen Future (http://www.ourstolenfuture.org)

Pesticide Action Network. "Many U.S. Residents Carry Toxic Pesticides Above 'Safe' Levels," http://www.panna.org, May 11, 2004.

"Pesticide Facts," Real Alternatives to Toxins in the Environment (http://www.chebucto.ns.ca)

"Range of Jobs Tied to Degenerative Brain Disease," *Reuters,* August 18, 2005.

Robbins, John. *Diet For a New America.* New World Library, 1987.

Rogers, Sherry A. *Chemical Sensitivity.* Keats Good Health Guide, 1995.

Schettler, Ted; Solomon, Gina; Valenti, Maria; and Huddle, Annette. *Generations at Risk.* MIT Press, 2000.

Schlosser, Eric. *Fast Food Nation.* HarperCollins, 2002.

Schwartz, John. "Causes of ALS still unknown," *The New York Times,* March 8, 2005.

Sheppard, Jane. "Has the Cause of Crib Death (SIDS) Been Found?" Healthy Child (http://healthychild.com).

Simons, Paul. "Can you dig it?" *Guardian,* May 22, 2004.

Simontacchi, Carol. *The Crazy Makers.* Tarcher, 2001.

Spears, Tom. "Flawed Tests Hide Pesticide Danger," *Ottawa Citizen,* September 30, 2001.

"Test Find High Mercury Levels In Fish," *Associated Press,* September 15, 2005.

Williams, Rose Marie. "More on 'inert,'" *Townsend Letter for Doctors and Patients,* July 2004.

Winter, MS, Ruth. *Vitamin E.* Three Rivers Press, 1998.

Yurkovsky, Savely. "Multiple Chemical Sensitivity ... From Treatments to Cure," *Townsend Letter for Doctors and Patients,* January 2001.

Chapter Three: A History of the Hundred-Year Lie

Abramson, John. *Overdosed America.* HarperCollins, 2004.

Atkins, Robert C. *Dr. Atkins' Age-Defying Diet Revolution.* St. Martin's Press, 2000.

Baillie-Hamilton, Paula. *Toxic Overload.* Penguin, 2005.

Blaylock, Russell. *Excitotoxins.* Health Press, 1997.

Bryson, Christopher. *The Fluoride Deception.* Seven Stories Press, 2004.

"Chemical Coating May Cause Cancer," Knight-Ridder Newspapers, June 29, 2005.

Colborn, Theo; Dumanoski, Dianne; and Myers, John. *Our Stolen Future.* Plume, 1997.

Cone, Marla. "Report: EPA Failing to Study Chemicals' Health Risks." *Los Angeles Times,* July 13, 2005.

De Graf, John; Wann, David; and Naylor, Thomas H. *Affluenza.* Berrett-Koehler Publishers, 2001.

"FDA Warns About ADHD Drug Strattera." *Associated Press,* September 29, 2005.

Fischer, Joannie. "The Molding of the World: Once the Butt of Jokes, Plastics Have Infiltrated Every Corner of Modern Life." *U.S. News,* June 25, 2001.

Fox, Maggie. "Half of Bankruptcy Due to Medical Bills." *Reuters,* February 2, 2005.

Fried, Stephen. *Bitter Pills.* Bantam Books, 1998.

Garrett, Laurie. *The Coming Plague.* Penguin Books, 1994.

Gold, Mark D. "The Bitter Truth About Artificial Sweeteners." *Nexus Magazine,* vol. 2, no. 28 (Oct–Nov 1995) and vol. 3, no. 1 (Dec 1995–Jan 1996).

Graedon, Joe and Graedon, Teresa. *Dangerous Drug Interactions.* St. Martin's Press, 1999.

Harris, Gardiner. "FDA Puts New Regulations on Severe-Acne Treatment." *The New York Times,* August 13, 2005.

Krimsky, Sheldon. *Hormonal Chaos.* Johns Hopkins University Press, 2000.

Liberman, Shari and Bruning, Nancy. *The Real Vitamin & Mineral Book.* Penguin, 1997.

McTaggart, Lynne. *What Doctors Don't Tell You.* Avon Books, 1996.

"More Men Seek Breast Reduction." *The Sunday Times,* July 31, 2005.

National Academies. "Major Advances in Biology Should Be Used to Assess Birth Defects From Toxic Chemicals." www4.nationalacademies.org, June 1, 2000.

Nestle, Marion. *Safe Food.* University of California Press, 2003.

Olmsted, Dan. "The Age of Autism: Mercury Goes to Work." *Science Daily,* October 17, 2005.

"Paxil Alert For Pregnant Women." *The New York Times,* September 29, 2005.

"The Public Images of Chemistry in the Twentieth Century: List of Abstracts." International Conference, Paris, September 17–18, 2004.

Robbins, John. *Diet For a New America.* New World Library, 1987.

Robbins, John. *The Food Revolution.* Conari Press, 2001.

Sarjeant, Doris and Evans, Karen. *Hard to Swallow: The Truth about Food Additives.* Alive Books, Burnaby, B.C., 1999.

Sax, Leonard. "Ritalin: Better Living Through Chemistry?" World and I (http://www.worldandi.com, 2003).

Schettler, Ted; Solomon, Gina; Valenti, Maria; and Huddle, Annette. *Generations at Risk.* MIT Press, 2000.

"Study: New Diabetes Pill Deemed Dangerous." *Associated Press,* October 20, 2005.

"Vioxx, Celebrex May Be Overprescribed." *Reuters,* January 21, 2005.

Chapter Four: Wizards of Oz: The Food Industry

Animal Protection Institute. "What's Really in Pet Food," http://api4animals.org

Baillie-Hamilton, Paula. *Toxic Overload.* Penguin, 2005.

Belfield, Wendell O. "Food Not Fit for a Pet." http://belfield.com

Blaylock, Russell. *Excitotoxins.* Health Press, 1997.

Borenstein, Seth. "Traces of Toxic Chemicals Found in Supermarket Food." Knight-Ridder Newspapers, September 2, 2004.

Bourland, Charles T. "Challenges for Space Food Systems." *NASA FTCSC News,* December 2004.

Carter, Meg. "Nature gets a hand . . . ." http://www.timesonline.co.uk, August 13, 2005.

Castel, Frédéric. "A Gastronomical Treat for Discovery's Crew," http://www.space.com, December 15, 1999.

Center for Science in the Public Interest. "CSPI's Guide to Food Additives." http://www.cspinet.org

Colborn, Theo; Dumanoski, Dianne; and Myers, John. *Our Stolen Future.* Plume, 1997.

Cordain, Loren. *The Paleo Diet.* John Wiley & Sons, 2002.

Critser, Greg. *Fat Land.* Houghton-Mifflin, 2003.

"The Dark Side of Recycling." *NEXUS Magazine,* vol. 4, no. 1, Dec '96–Jan '97.

DeGelia, Frances. "Pet Food: Nutrition or Nightmare?" *The Touchstone,* vol. IX, no. 1, Feb/Mar 1999.

De Graf, John; Wann, David; and Naylor, Thomas H. *Affluenza.* Berrett-Koehler Publishers, 2001.

Dodds, W. Jean. "Including Homemade and Raw Fed Diets," *Issues in Nutrition* (http://canine-epilepsy.com).

"Eating Dirt: It Might Be Good For You," ABC News, October 3, 2005.

Enig, Mary and Fallon, Sally. "The Oiling of America," *Nexus Magazine*, vol. 6, no. 1, Dec 1998-Jan 1999.

Environmental Working Group. "Farm Runoff, Chlorination By-products, and Human Health," http://ewg.org, January 8, 2002.

_____ "Pesticides in Produce," http://FoodNews.org

_____ "Rocket Fuel in Drinking Water," http://ewg.org/reports

Farhi, Paul. "The Man Who Gave America a Taste of the Future," http://www.washington post.com, July 22, 2005.

Food and Drug Administration. "Recommendations for Submission of Chemical and Technological Data for Direct Food Additive and GRAS Food Ingredient Petitions," Center for Food Safety and Applied Nutrition (http://www.cfsan.fda.gov), May 1993.

Fritz, Bob. "Dog Food Exposed," http://www.fila.org

Gertner, Jon. "Eat Chocolate, Live Longer?" *The New York Times Magazine*, October 10, 2004.

Ginsberg, Debra. "Sweet, but Sinister," http://www.organicstyle.com, June 2005.

Goettlich, Paul. "Get Plastic Out of Your Diet," http://www.mindfully.org, November 16, 2003.

Gold, Mark D. "The Bitter Truth About Artificial Sweeteners," *Nexus Magazine*, vol. 2, no. 28 (Oct-Nov 1995) and vol. 3, no. 1 (Dec 1995–Jan 1996).

Granby, Kit and Vahl, Martin. "Investigation of the Herbicide Glyphosate and the Plant Growth Regulators Chlormequat and Mepiquat in Cereals Produced in Denmark," *Food Additives and Contaminants*, vol. 18, no. 10, October 2001.

Huber, Gary. "Foods That May Cause Migraine Headaches," *Tyler Morning Telegraph*, March 9, 2005.

Hull, Janet Starr. "Food Additives to Avoid," http://www.sweetpoison.com

Human Adaptation and Countermeasures Office. "Nutritional Biochemistry Overview," http://haco.jsc.nasa.gov, September 24, 1999.

International Food Information Council. "Food Additives," http://www.ific.org, August 2000.

International Food Information Council. "Food Ingredients," http://www.ific.org, May 2004.

Jha, Alok. "Close Encounters." *The Guardian*, May 22, 2004.

Kallen, Ben. "Clear Water." *Natural Health*, July/August 2004.

Kennedy, Ron. "Addiction to Sugar," The Doctor's Medical Library (http://medical-library.net), 2005.

_____ *The Thinking Person's Guide to Perfect Health*, Context Publications, CA, 1996.

Korten, David C. *The Post-Corporate World*. Kumarion Press, 1999.

Legal Information Institute. "Food Additives." www.law.cornell.edu, August 18, 2005.

Levenstein, Harvey. *Revolution at the Table*. University of California Press, 2003.

Loecher, Barbara. "Is Your Water Fit to Drink?" *Prevention*, April 2004.

Martin, Ann. *Food Pets Die For: Shocking Facts About Pet Food*. NewSage Press, 1997.

Meléndez, Mel. "Arizona Issues Ban On Harmful Candies." *The Arizona Republic*, August 14, 2005.

Miller, Karen and Phillips, Tony. "Altered Gravity Plays an Unexpected Role in Obesity and Weight Loss." Science@NASA (http://www.nasa.gov).

"MSG is Sometimes Hidden in Food Labels," http://www.truthinlabeling.org

Ness, Carol. "Fighting for the Future of Food." *San Francisco Chronicle*, November 7, 2004.

Nestle, Marion. *Food Politics*. University of California Press, 2002.

Nestle, Marion. *Safe Food*. University of California Press, 2003.

Newcombe, Rachel. "Is Junk Food Addictive?" http://bupa.co.uk, July 19, 2003.

Noguchi, Soichi. "Space Food Tasting." Japan Aerospace Exploration Agency (http://sts-114.jaxa.jp), 2004.

Northwest Environment Watch. "Flame Retardants in Puget Sound Residents." http://northwestwatch.org, February 2004.

"Nutrition Challenges During Space Travel." http://www.medicinalfoodnews.com/vol06/issue3.

"Obesity," truthinlabeling.org

"Pesticides May Do Away with Us Long Before They Kill Off the Insects We Hate," Newsinferno.com, August 17, 2005.

"The Pet Food Industry and its Questionable Practices," *NEXUS Magazine*, vol. 10, no. 5, Aug–Sept 2003.

Pitcairn, Richard H. and Pitcairn, Susan Hubble. *Natural Health for Dogs and Cats*, Rodale Press, 1995.

Powers, Barbara. "Diet for a Small Pet." *Consumer News*, 2002.

Price, DDS, and Weston A. *Nutrition and Physical Degeneration*. Price-Pottenger, 1939.

Rabin, Roni. "Study Finds Link Between Fries and Breast Cancer." Newsday.com, August 18, 2005.

Rappole, Clinton L.; Bourland, Charles T.; and Vodovotz, Yael. "Design of a Food Service and Food Processing System for Long-Duration Missions in a Closed Environment." Institute for Space Systems Operations (http://isso.uh.edu), 1996.

Redstone, Michael. "NASA Astronaut Gives Summer Camp Students a Lesson in Outer Space." Missoulian.com, July 20, 2004.

Robbins, John. *The Food Revolution*. Conari Press, 2001.

Roderick, Kyle. "Filtration and Purification." *Natural Health*, July/Aug 2004.

Sarjeant, Doris and Evans, Karen. *Hard to Swallow: The Truth about Food Additives*. Alive Books, Burnaby, B.C., 1999.

Schafer, Kristin S.; Reeves, Margaret; Spitzer, Skip; and Kegley, Susan E. "Chemical Trespass," Pesticide Action Network, May 2004.

Schettler, Ted; Solomon, Gina; Valenti, Maria; and Huddle, Annette. *Generations at Risk*. MIT Press, 2000.

Schlichenmeyer, Terri. "10 Foods That (Thankfully) Flopped," http://mentalfloss.com.

Schlick, Greg and Bubenheim, David L. *Quinoa: Candidate Crop for NASA's Controlled Ecological Life Support Systems*. ASHA Press, 1996.

Schlosser, Eric. *Fast Food Nation*. HarperCollins, 2002.

Science@NASA. "Leafy Green Astronauts," http://science.nasa.gov, April 9, 2001.

Science@NASA. "Space Seeds Return to Earth." http://science.nasa.gov, July 25, 2001.

Sellman, Sherrill. "Drugs and Chemicals Straight from the Tap." *Nexus*, May–June 2005.

Senter, Carlin. "Weightlessness and Weight Loss: Malnutrition in Space." *Nutrition Noteworthy*, vol. 4, issue 1, article 6, 2001.

Severson, Kim. "Turning the Tables on America's Diet," *San Francisco Chronicle*, August 12, 2004.

Shapira, Jacob. "Food Synthesis by Physicochemical Methods," http://history.nasa.gov.

Sharp, Renee and Lunder, Sonya. "Suspect Salads: Toxic Rocket Fuel Found in Samples of Winter Lettuce." Environmental Working Group, 2003.

Sheftel, Victor O. "Harmful Substances in Plastics." http://www.mindfully.org, 2000.

Shiga, David. "The Zero Gravity Diet." Science News Online, vol. 167, no. 11, March 12, 2005.

Simontacchi, Carol. *The Crazy Makers*. Tarcher, 2001.

Smith, Gar. "A Look Inside a Rendering Plant." *NEXUS Magazine*, vol. 4, no. 1, Dec 1996–Jan 1997.

Smith, Jeffrey M. *Seeds of Deception*. Yes! Books, 2003.

Smith, Scott M. "Nutrition for Space Exploration." http://www.dsls.usra.edu.

Snyder, Amy. "Plant-Based Life Support in Space." http://www.rso.cornell.edu.

Stevens, Jane Ellen. "Bumpy Road to Mars." *Smithsonian Magazine* (smithsonianmag.si.edu), June 2004.

"Take It From a Vet," *Alternative Medicine*. September 2004.

Tou, Janet et al. "Evaluation of NASA Foodbars as a Standard Diet for Use in Short-Term Rodent Space Flight Studies." ScienceDirect.com, *Nutrition*, vol. 19, issues 11–12, Nov–Dec 2003.

"The Truth About Cats and Dogs," *NEXUS Magazine*, vol. 4, no. 1, December 1996.

"Veggie Nutrients Dip in Test." *Omaha World-Herald*, January 29, 2000.

Vodovotz, Yael; Bourland, Charles T.; and Rappole, Clinton L. "Advanced Life Support Food Development: A New Challenge," http://www.transorbital.net

Wahlberg, David. "America's Melting Pot is Bubbling Over with Fat." Cox News Service, December 15, 2004.

Warner, Melanie. "Science's Quest to Banish Fat in Tasty Ways." http://www.nytimes.com, August 11, 2005.

Warner, Melanie. "US: Senomyx's Fake Flavors." *The New York Times*, April 6, 2005.

Watts, Geoff. "The Devil in their Diet." Independent.co.uk, August 16, 2004.

Williamson, David. "Study: Water Purification with Chlorine Poses No Threat to Pregnant Women." http://www.foodconsumer.org, July 31, 2005.

Chapter Five: Sorcerer's Apprentices: The Drug and Medical Industries

Abramson, John. *Overdosed America*. HarperCollins, 2004.

Acuff, Robert V. "Synthetic vs. Natural Vitamin E." *Nature's Impact* magazine.

Angell, Marcia. *The Truth About the Drug Companies*. Random House, 2004.

Associated Press. "Mercury in Children's Vaccines Worried Merck Execs." *The Press Democrat,* February 9, 2005.

Atkins, Robert C. *Dr. Atkins' Age-Defying Diet Revolution.* St. Martin's Press, 2000.

Ausubel, Kenny. *Ecological Medicine.* Sierra Club Books, 2004.

"Avoidance of Toxic and Unhealthy Exposures." http://www.holisticmed.com

Avorn, Dr. Jerry. *Powerful Medicines.* Knopf, 2004.

Baillie-Hamilton, Paula. *Toxic Overload.* Penguin, 2005.

Barkee, Michael. *Politically Incorrect Nutrition.* Vital Health Publishing, 2004.

Bates, David W. "Rx Dangers." *Bottom Line Health.* September 2004.

Blaylock, Russell L. "The Truth Behind the Vaccine Coverup." http://mercola.com.

Blumenthal, Mark. "Many Herbs and Drugs Don't Mix." *Bottom Line Health.* November 2004.

Brownlee, Shannon. "Health, Hope and Hype." http://www.washingtonpost.com, August 3, 2003.

Bryson, Christopher. *The Fluoride Deception.* Seven Stories Press, 2004.

Cavallo, Jo. "Drugs That Don't Mix," *Family Circle.* March 4, 2003.

Cohen, Jay S. *Over Dose.* Tarcher, 2001.

"The Color of Money." Health Sciences Institute e-Alert.

"Colo. Scientists Find Chemicals in Waters." start.earthlink.net, January 19, 2005.

Connett, Paul. "The Absurdities of Water Fluoridation." *Nexus New Times* (http://www.nexusmagazine.com), Nov–Dec 2004.

"Cows Dropping Poisonous Poop." Newswires, September 2, 2001.

"Dr. Berman's Sex Rx." *The Los Angeles Times,* October 2, 2005.

Feher, Miklos and Schmidt, Jonathan M. "Differences Between Drugs, Natural Products, and Molecules from Combinatorial Chemistry." American Chemical Society, 2002.

"Fluoridation Chemicals." Second Look (http://www.slweb.org).

Fluoride Action Network. "Facts About Fluoridation." http://www.fluoridealert.org, March 2002.

"Foster Kids on Mind-Altering Drugs?" http://www.woai.com, November 2004.

Freudenheim, Milt. "Drug Prices For Elderly Surge Ahead in America." *The New York Times,* August 17, 2005.

Fried, Stephen. *Bitter Pills.* Bantam Books, 1998.

Gardner, Amanda. "More Than 2.5 Million US Kids Medicated for ADHD." *HealthDay News,* September 1, 2005.

Garrett, Laurie. *The Coming Plague.* Penguin Books, 1994.

Golan, David. "Building Better Medicines." *Newsweek,* Summer 2005.

Gordon, Serena. "Antioxidant Levels May Be Linked to Autism." *HealthDay,* http://www.forbes.com, April 3, 2005.

Graedon, Joe and Graedon, Teresa. *Dangerous Drug Interactions.* St. Martin's Press, 1999.

Hays, Carl. "Against the Dental Establishment." American Council on Science and Health (http://www.acsh.org), June 13, 2002.

Jefferson, David J. "America's Most Dangerous Drug." *Newsweek,* August 8, 2005.

Kelley, Raina. "How to Quit the Cure." *Newsweek,* August 6, 2005.

Kennedy, Ron. *The Thinking Person's Guide to Perfect Health.* Context Publications, 1996.

Konner, Melvin. *Medicine at the Crossroads.* Pantheon, 1993.

Leibovitch, Eric R. "Food-Drug Dangers." *Bottom Line Health,* October 2004.

Lieberman, Shari and Bruning, Nancy. *The Real Vitamin & Mineral Book.* Penguin, 1997.

Lidsky, Theodore and Schneider, Jay. *Brain Candy.* Simon & Schuster, 2001.

Limeback, Hardy. "Why I Am Now Officially Opposed to Adding Fluoride to Drinking Water." Second Look (http://www.slweb.org), April 2000.

Masters, Roger D. "Silicofluorides and Higher Blood Lead." Second Look (slweb.org), June 17, 2001.

Mokhiber, Russell and Weissman, Robert. "Stripping Away Big Pharma's Figleaf." AlterNet.org, June 17, 2002.

Nano, Stephanie. "Daily multivitamins found to cut AIDS risk in half." *Associated Press,* July 1, 2004.

National Treasury Employees Union. "Why EPA's Headquarters Professionals' Union Opposes Fluoridation." Second Look (http://www.slweb.org), May 1, 1999.

"Natural E vs. Synthetic." *Townsend Letter for Doctors & Patients,* July 1999.

Nickell, Joe. "Peddling Snake Oil." Committee for the Scientific Investigation of Claims of the Paranormal (http://www.csicop.org), December 1998.

"Not In My Water Supply." *Time,* October 24, 2005.

Null, Gary et al. "Death by Medicine." LE Magazine (http://www.lef.org), March 2004.

Pratley, Nils. "Bitter Pill for the World's Drug Companies." *The Guardian,* September 12, 2003.

Pringle, Evelyn. "Cut the Crap." http://www.stclairrecord.com, August 6, 2005.

"Report Shows Dental Cavities Declining Among Children." *Baltimore Sun,* October 2, 2005.

Robbins, John. *Reclaiming Our Health.* Kramer, 1998.

Rubin, Jordan S. *Patient, Heal Thyself.* Freedom Press, 2003.

Sax, Leonard. "Ritalin: Better Living Through Chemistry?" http://www.worldandi.com, 2003.

Schneider, Andrew. "New EPA Rules on Human Test Subjects." *Baltimore Sun,* September 15, 2005.

Seavey, Todd; Hays, Carl; and Dodes, John E. "Fluoride and Amalgam Debate." American Council on Science and Health (http://www.acsh.org), June 13, 2002.

Sinclair, Wayne and Pressinger, Richard. "Chemicals and Effects Upon Health," http://www.chem-tox.com.

Treadway, Scott. "The Naturally Occurring Paradigm."

Vanderhaeghe, Lorna and Bouic, Patrick. *The Immune System Cure.* Prentice-Hall, 1999.

"Vitamin E Might Make Heart Disease Worse." *Associated Press,* November 10, 2004.

Wallach, Joel D. and Lan, Ma. *Rare Earths, Forbidden Cures.* Double Happiness, 1996.

Winter, MS, Ruth. *Vitamin E.* Three Rivers Press, 1998.

Chapter Six: Are We Becoming a Mutant Species?

Alexander, Richard. "Birth Defects in Children of Workers Exposed to Chemicals." http://www.consumerlawpage.com

Algalita Marine Research Foundation. "Plastic Generation and Recovery Graph 1960–1995." http://mindfully.org.

American Council on Science and Health. "Biomonitoring: Measuring Levels of Chemicals in People—and What the Results Mean." http://acsh.org/publications, August 2005.

American Museum of Natural History. "Scientific Experts Believe We Are in the Midst of the Fastest Mass Extinction in Earth's History." http://www.amnh.org

Baillie-Hamilton, Paula. *Toxic Overload*. Penguin, 2005.

BBC News. "Poisons May Pass Down Generations." http://newsvote.bbc.co.uk

——— "Traffic Damages Male Fertility."

——— "Traffic Fumes Damage Human DNA."

Begley, Sharon. "How a Second, Secret Genetic Code Turns Genes On and Off," *The Wall Street Journal*, July 23, 2004.

——— "Mom's Care Can Alter DNA in Her Offspring," *The Wall Street Journal*, July 16, 2004.

——— "Lab Mice Take After Mom's Diet." *The Wall Street Journal*, August 15, 2003.

Blackless, Melanie et al. "How Sexually Dimorphic Are We?" *American Journal of Human Biology*, 2000.

Blakeslee, Sandra. "A Pregnant Mother's Diet May Turn the Genes Around," *The New York Times*, October 7, 2003.

Boggan, Steve. "Is My Baby a Boy? Is My Baby a Girl? No One Could Tell Me." Times Online.co.uk, July 26, 2005.

Briggs, Helen. " 'Gender-bender' Fish problem Widens," BBC News Online, September 6, 2000.

Burne, Jerome. "Animal Testing is a Disaster." *Guardian*, May 24, 2001.

Buttram, MD, Harold E.; Kreider, RN, Susan; Yurko, Alan R. "Vaccines and Genetic Mutation." freeyurko.bizland.com/vacgen.html, October 11, 2002.

ChemicalIndustryArchives.org. "People vary enormously in their reactions to toxic substances." http://www.chemicalarchives.com

Colborn, Theo; Dumanoski, Dianne; and Myers, John. *Our Stolen Future*. Plume, 1997.

Cone, Marla. "Abnormalities in Fish off L.A. Coast." *Los Angeles Times*, November 13, 2005.

Connor, Steve. "Man-Made Pesticides Blamed for Fall in Male Fertility Over Past 50 Years." Independent/UK, June 3, 2005.

Cowan, Robert C. "The Downstream Dangers of Your Perfume," *Christian Science Monitor*, December 20, 2004.

Cummins, Joe and Ho, Mae-Wan. "Atrazine Poisoning Worse Than Suspected." Institute of Science in Society (http://i-sis.org.uk).

De Graf, John; Wann, David; and Naylor, Thomas H. *Affluenza*. Berrett-Koehler Publishers, 2001.

"Diesel Gases Masculinize Fetal Rodents." *Science News,* January 20, 2001.

Eldredge, Niles. "The Sixth Extinction." ActionBioscience.org, June 2001.

"Emerging Science on the Impacts of Endocrine Disruptors on the Immune System and Disease Resistance," http://Our StolenFuture.org

EurekAlert. "Genetic Mutations Linked to Practice of Burning Coal in Homes in China," http://www.eurekalert.org, September 30, 2004.

Gardner, Amanda. "Pesticides Cause Lasting Damage to Rats' Sperm," *Forbes,* June 2, 2005.

Greek, C. Ray and Greek, Jean Swingle. *Specious Science: Why Experiments on Animals Harm Humans.* Continuum Publishing Group, 2003.

GreenBiz.com. "Chemical Industry's Product Responsibility Still in Short Supply." September 7, 2005.

Hayes, T.B. et al. "Hermaphroditic, Demasculinized Frogs after Exposure to the Herbicide, Atrazine at Low Ecologically Relevant Doses." http://OurStolenFuture.org.

Henderson, Mark. "Junk Medicine: Chemical Hysteria." Times Online, July 30, 2005.

Hunter, Philip. "Toxins Harm Descendant Fertility." The-Scientist.com, June 6, 2005.

Kirby, Alex. "Pollution damages intelligence," BBC News Sci/Tech (news.bbc.co.uk/1/hi/sci/tech).

Kotulak, Ronald. "Studies: Brain's Evolution Not Over." *Chicago Tribune,* September 9, 2005.

Krimsky, Sheldon. *Hormonal Chaos.* Johns Hopkins University Press, 2000.

Landrigan, Philip; Garg, Anjali; and Droller, Daniel B.J. "Assessing the Effects of Endocrine Disruptors in the National Children's Study," *Environmental Health Perspectives,* vol. 111, no. 13, October 2003.

Larsen, Janet. "The Sixth Great Extinction," Earth Policy Institute, March 2, 2004.

LeBlanc, Gerald A. "Assessing Deleterious Ecosystem-level Effects of Environmental Pollutants as a Means of Avoiding Evolutionary Consequences," *Environmental Health Perspectives,* Vol. 102, #3, March 1994.

Lemonick, Michael. "Could Toxin Damage Become Hereditary?" *Time* Online, June 3, 2005.

Lovett, Richard A. "Toxicologists Brace for Genomics Revolution," *Science,* vol. 289, issue 5479, July 2000.

Lovgren, Stefan. "Low Sperm Counts Blamed on Pesticides in U.S. Water." *National Geographic News,* April 27, 2005.

"The Lowdown on Low-Dose Endocrine Disruptors." *Environmental Health Perspectives* (http://www.ehpnet1.niehs.nih.gov), vol. 109, no. 9, September 2001.

Miller, Henry I. "Halting the March of Unreason, Including Organic Foods." *San Francisco Chronicle,* May 14, 2005.

Miner, John. "Drop in Male Births Raises Serious Fears." *London Free Press,* August 19, 2005.

Montague, Tim. "A New Way to Inherit Environmental Harm." *Rachel's Environment & Health News,* June 9, 2005.

Moore, Charles. "Great Pacific Garbage Patch." *Santa Barbara News-Press,* October 27, 2002.

———— "Plastic is Drastic: World's Largest 'Landfill' is in the Middle of the Ocean." Algalita Marine Research Foundation, November 1, 2002.

"More Men Seek Breast Reduction." *The Sunday Times,* July 31, 2005.

National Academies. "Major Advances in Biology Should be Used to Assess Birth Defects from Toxic Chemicals." http://www4.nationalacademies.org, June 1, 2000.

Olsen, Geary W. et al. "Historical Comparison of Perfluorooctanesulfonate, Perfluorooctanoate and other Fluorochemicals in Human Blood." *Environmental Health Perspectives,* Vol. 113, no. 5, May 2005.

Our Stolen Future (http://www.ourstolenfuture.org).

———— "Changes in Human Sex Ratio."

———— "New findings on the timing of sexual maturity."

———— "The Science of sperm count declines."

———— "Scientific findings of the impacts of endocrine disruptors at low doses."

Palumbi, Stephen R. "Humans as the World's Greatest Evolutionary Force." http://www.sciencemag.org, vol. 293, no. 5536, September 2001.

Paulson, Tom. "Startling Study on Toxins' Harm." *Seattle-Post Intelligencer,* June 3, 2005.

Pelton, Tom. "Drug traces found in water pose problem for wildlife." *Baltimore Sun,* October 17, 2005.

Raloff, Janet. "That Feminine Touch: Are Men Suffering From Prenatal or Childhood Exposures to 'Hormonal' Toxicants?" *Science News,* January 22, 1994.

Rapp, Doris J. *Our Toxic World.* Environmental Medical Research Foundation, 2004.

Rudel, Ruthann A. et al. "Phthalates, Alkylphenols, Pesticides, Polybrominated Diphenyl Ethers, and other Endocrine-Disrupting Compounds in Indoor Air and Dust." *Environmental Science & Technology,* September 13, 2003.

Schettler, Ted et al. "How Environmental Toxins May Effect Reproductive Health in Massachusetts." Greater Boston Physicians for Social Responsibility and Massachusetts Public Interest Research Group.

Sellman, Sherrill. "The Problem of Precocious Puberty." *Nexus Magazine,* vol. 11, no. 3, Apr–May 2004.

Shiga, David. "Where Did all the Baby Boys Go?" NewScientist.com, September 5, 2005.

Skinner, Michael K. "Study Summary." *Science,* June 3, 2005.

Stier, Jeff. "Biomonitoring and Body Burden in Perspective." American Council on Science and Health (http://www.acsh.org), July 21, 2005.

"Surprising Study Shows Role of Toxins in Inherited Disease." Washington State University News Service, June 2, 2005.

Trosko, James E. and Zacharewski, Timothy R. "Project 8: Epigenetic Effects of Pre- and Post Remediated Environmental Toxicants. . . ." http://www.iet.msu.edu/NIEHS_Sfund/Project8.htm

Vince, Gaia. "Pregnant Smokers Increase Grandkids' Asthma Risk." *New Scientist,* April 12, 2005.

Waldman, Peter. "From an Ingredient in Cosmetics, Toys, A Safety Concern." *The Wall Street Journal,* October 4, 2005.

Weise, Elizabeth. "Chemicals in Everyday Goods Disrupt Hormones." *USA Today,* August 3, 2005.

――――― "Damage from Toxins Can Pass to Offspring." USAToday.com

Weiss, Rick. " 'Data Quality' Law is Nemesis of Regulation," http://www.washington post.com, August 16, 2004.

Yang, Chun-Yuh. "Association Between Petrochemical Air Pollution and Adverse Pregnancy Outcomes in Taiwan." *Archives of Environmental Health,* Sept–Oct 2002.

Chapter Seven: Our Health Is Naturally Occurring

Airola, Paavo O. "Nutrition Wisdom." http://www.gentlebirth.org

All-Natural.com. "The Ultimate Secret to Long Life." *Scientific American,* January 1996.

Angell, Marcia. *The Truth About the Drug Companies.* Random House, 2004.

Anti-Ageing US. "Anti-Aging Medicine," anti-ageing.us

Ausubel, Kenny. *Ecological Medicine.* Sierra Club Books, 2004.

――――― *Nature's Operating Instructions.* Sierra Club Books, 2004.

Avorn, Jerry. *Powerful Medicines.* Knopf, 2004.

Baillie-Hamilton, Paula. *Toxic Overload.* Penguin, 2005.

Bass, Stanley S. "In Search of the Ultimate Vegetarian Diet." http://www.drbass.com.

BBC News. "Dieting Hope for Monastic Elixir." http://www.bbc.co.uk, August 30, 2005.

BBC News. "Positive Thinking a Pain Reliever." http://www.bbc.co.uk, September 5, 2005.

Benson, Herbert. *Timeless Healing.* Scribner, 1996.

Bieler, Henry G. *Food Is Your Best Medicine.* Random House, 1966.

"Bioprospecting: Medicine Quest" (interview with Mark J. Plotkin), http://www.action bioscience.org, October 2000.

Bower, B. "Elderly Helpers Have Longevity Advantage." *Science News.* July 26, 2003.

"Brain scan reveal placebo effect in depressed patients," http://www.newscientist.com, January 2, 2002.

Brown, Walter A. "The Best Medicine?" *Psychology Today.* September 1997.

Carper, Jean. *Food—Your Miracle Medicine.* HarperCollins, 1993.

"Chromium Picolinate Linked with Reduced Carbohydrate Cravings in People With Atypical Depression," *Journal of Psychiatric Practice,* September 29, 2005.

Cohen, Jay S. *Over Dose.* Tarcher, 2001.

Consumers Union. "Organic Foods Really DO Have Less Pesticides." http://www.common dreams.org, May 8, 2002.

"Corn grain mould used as pesticide." EurekAlert!, August 8, 2005.

Corning, Peter. *Nature's Magic.* Cambridge University Press, 2003.

Crowther, Penny. "Organic Food, Farming, and Family Health." http://www.familiesonline.co.uk, May 13, 2001.

Davis, Jeanie Lerch. "Add a Decade to Your Life." WebMD Medical News (my.webmd.com), July 20, 2001.

"Dietary Supplements Slash Prisoners' Antisocial Acts." *Crime Times,* vol. 8, no. 3, 2002.

Duke, James A. *The Green Pharmacy.* Rodale Press, 1997.

Foltz-Gray, Dorothy. "The Magic of Mushrooms." *Alternative Medicine,* Jan/Feb 2003.

Ford, Norman D. "Where People Live Longest and Why." http://www.nohypehealth.org

Fujimori, Leila. "Okinawans Chew Way to the Top of Longevity Charts," http://www.starbulletin.com, July 30, 2001.

Gavrilov, Leonid A. "Life Extension, Caloric Restriction, and Scientific Philanthropy." Science Advisory Board (http://www.scienceboard.net).

Gavrilova, Natalia S. and Gavrilov, Leonid A. "Search for Predictors of Exceptional Human Longevity." Society of Actuaries, 2005.

Geiger, Debbe. "Healthy Hints from Okinawa for Good Living Past 100." http://www.okinawaprogram.com, July 23, 2001.

Gower, Timothy. "Aging, Deferred," *Alternative Medicine,* June 2003.

Hall, Celia. "I've Seen Herbal Remedy Make Tumours Disappear, Says Respected Cancer Doctor," http://www.telegraph.co.uk/news, September 20, 2004.

"Health, Behaviour: It's All in the Food." *Guardian,* May 9, 2005.

Healy, Melissa. "Organic Questions." *Los Angeles Times,* October 19, 2004.

Himes, Christine L. "Age 100 and Counting." Population Reference Bureau (http://www.prb.org), April 2003.

International Longevity Center—USA. "The Secrets of Longevity Genes," June 1, 2004.

Jeune, Bernard. "In Search of the First Centenarians." http://www.demogr.mpg.de, March 2000.

Kamen, Betty. "Long-Lived Cultures and Calcium." http://www.nutricology.com/news/letters

Kilham, Chris. "Horny Goat Weed: More Than Just a Name." http://www.health.discovery.com, 2005.

Kinderlehrer, Jane. "Death Rides a Slow Bus in Hunza." http://www.worldwithoutcancer.com

Koenig, Robert. "Sardinia's Mysterious Male Methuselahs." *Science,* vol. 291, issue 5511, March 16, 2001.

Konner, Melvin. *Medicine at the Crossroads.* Pantheon, 1993.

"Longevity," *Men's Health,* September 2004.

Maine Organic Farmers and Gardeners Association. "Why Certified Organic Food Is Better Food," http://www.mofga.org

"Modern Methuselahs," http://www.custance.org, May 14, 1997.

Murray, Christopher. "Japan Number One in New 'Healthy Life' System." http://www.who.int.

"National Longevity Recordholders." http://www.en.wikipedia.org, 2005.

Nestle, Marion. *Food Politics.* University of California Press, 2002.

Norton, Amy. "Going Raw: Better for Your Body?" http://www.msm.com.

Okinawa Centenarian Study. "Evidence-Based Gerontology." http://www.okinawaprogram.com.

Okinawa International Conference on Longevity. "Okinawa Longevity/Ageing is Uniquely a Celebration of Life!" http://www.oic-longevity.wwma.net, April 2004.

"Organic Gets Even Better." *Alternative Medicine,* June 2003.

"Organic Veggies are Healthier," *Prevention Magazine,* April 2004.

Paterson, John. "Organic Food: Are There Any Benefits?" *Bottom Line Health,* October 2002.

Pelton, Ross. *Mind Food & Smart Pills.* Doubleday, 1989.

"Pharma's New Enemy: Clean Living." *Forbes,* November 29, 2004.

"Phytochemicals May Protect Cartilage, Prevent Pain in Joints." *Proceedings of the National Academy of Sciences,* Sept. 27, 2005.

"Placebos Effect Revealed in Calmed Brain Cells." http://www.newscientist.com, May 16, 2004.

"Placebo Produces Surprise Biological Effect." http://www.newscientist.com, August 9, 2001.

Plotkin, Mark J. *Medicine Quest.* Viking Penguin, 2000.

Pollan, Michael. "How Organic Is Corporate/Industrial Organic?" *The New York Times Magazine,* May 13, 2001.

Reid, Brian. "The Nocebo Effect: Placebo's Evil Twin." *The Washington Post,* April 30, 2002.

Robbins, John. *The Food Revolution.* Conari Press, 2001.

Rosenfeld, Isadore. "Help Your Body Protect Itself." *Parade,* May 1, 2005.

Saltus, Richard. "The Secret of Life." *The Boston Globe,* May 22, 2001.

"The Secrets of Hunza Water." Escape to Cybertown (http://www.cybertown.com).

"Study: Most doctors use placebos." *Jerusalem Post,* September 19, 2004.

Takayama, Hideko. "Newsweek Features Healthy Okinawa Diet." http://www.okinawa diet.com, June 1, 2004.

Thierry Souccar. "Legendary Centenarians: Are They for Real?" http://www.thierry souccar.com, September 2004.

Torassa, Ulysses. "Living Long and Prospering." *San Francisco Chronicle,* June 3, 2001.

Vanderhaeghe, Lorna and Bouic, Patrick. *The Immune System Cure.* Prentice-Hall, 1999.

Viegas, Jennifer. "Garlic's Potent Effects Revealed," http://www.discoverychannel.com, August 15, 2005.

Walker, Morton. "Found: Nature's Perfect Food," *Townsend Letter for Doctors and Patients,* 2001.

Wallechinsky, David and Wallace, Irving. "Hunza in Pakistan," *The People's Almanac,* 1975–1981.

Wallis, Claudia. "The Right (and Wrong) Way to Treat Pain," *Time,* February 28, 2005.

Weil, Andrew. "Natural Pest Defense," *Prevention Magazine,* April 2004.

Weissman, Beth. "Organic foods helped Lari White lose weight," *Woman's World,* August 23, 2005.

Wellness Letter. "Eat Like an Okinawan," berkeleywellness.com, September 2001.

Wiseman, Paul. "Fabric of a Long Life." http://www.usatoday.com/news/health, January 3, 2002.

Yanick, Paul. "Food and Supplementation Benefits and Risks in Carcinogenesis." *Townsend Letter for Doctors and Patients,* October 2001.

"Zinc diet reduces violence in youths." *Sunday Times,* July 1997.

Chapter Eight: When Western Medicine Fails

"Age-Old Cures, Like the Maggot, Get U.S. Hearing." *The New York Times,* August 25, 2005.

"Analysis of Anti-rotavirus Activity of Extract From Stevia." *Antiviral Research,* January 2001.

"Ancient Chinese remedy may provide new treatment for malaria." *Independent,* August 19, 2004.

"Ancient Secrets of Plants' Miracle Cures." *London Observer,* August 21, 2005.

Atkins, MD, Robert C. *Dr. Atkins' Age-Defying Diet Revolution.* St. Martin's Press, 2000.

Ausubel, Kenny. *Ecological Medicine.* Sierra Club Books, 2004.

Ausubel, Kenny. *Nature's Operating Instructions.* Sierra Club Books, 2004.

"Automatic Detention of Stevia Leaves." U.S. Food and Drug Administration, Feb. 2, 1996.

Baillie-Hamilton, Paula. *Toxic Overload.* Penguin, 2005.

BBC News. "Herbal Remedies Do Work." http://www.bbc.co.uk, Spetember 28, 2004.

"Biopiracy and Traditional Knowledge," *The Hindu,* May 20, 2001.

"Bioprospecting: Medicine Quest." http://www.actionbioscience.org, October 2000.

"Bioresources and Biopiracy." *Science,* May 1998.

Colborn, Theo; Dumanoski, Dianne; and Myers, John. *Our Stolen Future.* Plume, 1997.

Copulos, Milt. "It's the FDA, We're Here To Burn Your Books," *Regulation,* vol. 21, no. 4., 1998.

Daily, Gretchen C. *Nature's Services.* Island Press, 1997.

"Doctors Used to Dismiss Magnetic Therapy . . ." *Independent,* January 18, 2005.

Fitzgerald, Randall. "The Case of the Dizzy Dame." *Alternative Medicine,* January 2003.

————— "Diagnosis Denied." *Alternative Medicine,* June 2003.

"Folk Remedies That Really Work." *Bottom Line Health,* December 2003.

Garrett, J.T. *The Cherokee Herbal.* Bear & Company, 2003.

Graedon, Joe and Graedon, Teresa. *Dangerous Drug Interactions.* St. Martin's Press, 1999.

Helmich, Portland. "A Triumph Over Cancer." *Alternative Medicine,* September 2004.

Konner, Melvin. *Medicine at the Crossroads.* Pantheon, 1993.

Lidsky, Theodore and Schneider, Jay. *Brain Candy.* Simon & Schuster, 2001.

McTaggart, Lynne. *What Doctors Don't Tell You.* Avon Books, 1996.

Mullen, William. "Meds Today, in 2000 B.C. Surprisingly Comparable." *Chicago Tribune,* October 28, 2005.

"Pharmacy Island," *Newsweek,* special issue, Summer 2005.

"Pirates in the garden of India." *New Science,* October 1996.

Plotkin, Mark J. *Medicine Quest.* Viking Penguin, 2000.

Prostate, "Therapeutic potential of curcumin," June 2001.

"The Right Time For a Cure." *Newsweek,* special issue, Summer 2005.

Robbins, John. *Reclaiming Our Health.* Kramer, 1998.

"Tibetan Medicine Packed With Unusual Pharmaceutical Properties." http://www.chinadaily.com, August 18, 2004.

University of Washington. "Ancient Chinese Folk Remedy Packs Anti-Cancer Punch."
    October 14, 2004.
Winter, Ruth. *Vitamin E.* Three Rivers Press, 1998.

Chapter Nine: Bringing It All Home

ABC News. "Whistleblower Questions Safety of Food Packaging," November 18, 2005.
Associated Press. "DuPont Fined More Than $10 M Over Teflon," December 14, 2005.
Harris, Gardiner. "New Drug Points up Problems in Developing Cancer Cures," *The New York Times,* December 21, 2005.
Kolata, Gina. "Environment and Cancer: The Links Are Elusive," *The New York Times,* December 13, 2005.
National Cancer Institute. "SEER Cancer Statistics Review 1975–2002."
The National Coalition on Health Care, "Facts on the Cost of Health Care," www.nchc.org.
OurStolenFuture.org, Vallombrosa Consensus Statement on Environmental Contaminants, October 2005.

Postscript: More Evidence to Penetrate Our Denial

Ambrose, Sue Goetinck. "Diets of Rodents May Have Tainted Decades of Research." *The Dallas Morning News,* August 1, 2006.
Boseley, Sarah. "Danger: Chemical Hazards." *The Guardian* (London), November 9, 2006.
Davis, Dr. Devra. "Toxic Chemicals Don't Just Hurt Us in Big Doses." MSNBC.com, Feb. 15, 2007.
Duncan, David Ewing. "The Pollution Within." *National Geographic,* October 2006.
Fahrenthold, David. "Male Bass Across Region Found to Be Bearing Eggs." *The Washington Post,* September 6, 2006.
Lawrence, Felicity. "Omega-3, Junk Food and the Link Between Violence and What We Eat." *The Guardian* (London), October 17, 2006.
Royte, Elizabeth. "How Prescription Drugs Are Poisoning Our Waters." *OnEarth Magazine,* October 23, 2006.
"Special Issue Examines Effects of Emerging Contaminants." *Environmental Science & Technology,* American Chemical Society, December 1, 2006.

ACKNOWLEDGMENTS

Without Thomas Lefebvre and Terry Cafferty, the research and writing of this book would never have been possible. Thomas convinced me to take an interest in this subject matter and conceived the title of this book, then provided valuable insights and advice every step of the way. He became absolutely indispensable in the last stage of the research process. Terry provided crucial support and wise counsel throughout the nine months of preliminary research and beyond.

Shawnee Free Jones contributed significant research assistance and helped to generate important ideas, and Lynnzee Elze did an exacting job on the bibliography and the index. Dr. Scott Treadway created the toxins questionnaire and provided valuable support during every phase of the process. Other assistance was provided by Angelo Druda, Dr. Daniel Bouwmeester, and Dr. John Laseter.

Special thanks go to my literary agent, Bill Gladstone, and to Ming Russell and Maureen Maloney of his Waterside Productions staff. My appreciation goes to Brian Tart, publisher of Dutton, who promptly secured this project when it was made available, and also to my editor at Dutton, Julie Doughty, for playing "idea tennis" with me during the editing phase. Thank you to John Raatz and his team at The Visioneering Group in Los Angeles for the public relations campaign and to David Rippe for his Internet marketing efforts.

Thanks to Brian and Anna Maria Clement and their staff at the Hippocrates Health Institute in West Palm Beach, Florida, for making my three-week research stay there so enlightening. Greg and Allison Rodgers, owners of the Mountain High Coffee Shop and its adjoining bookstore, are to be commended for tolerating my presence through many long mornings of reading and writing.

I also would like to extend my gratitude to a group of dedicated women who have been pioneers in documenting the effects of synthetic chemicals on human and animal health—Rachel Carson, and the physicians Doris J. Rapp, Paula Baillie-Hamilton, and Sherry Rogers.

INDEX